Henk J. Klasen

History of Free Skin Grafting

Knowledge or Empiricism?

With a Contribution by Tom Gibson

With 44 Figures

Springer-Verlag
Berlin Heidelberg New York

Dr. Henk J. Klasen
Academisch Ziekenhuis, Oostersingel 59, 9700 RB Groningen, The Netherlands

ISBN 3-540-10802-5 Springer-Verlag Berlin Heidelberg New York
ISBN 0-387-10802-5 Springer-Verlag New York Heidelberg Berlin

Typesetting, Printing, and Binding: Konrad Triltsch, Würzburg
2124/3130-543210

Foreword

Amidst the innumerable articles and books on plastic and reconstructive surgery, a thorough and extensive study of the history of free skin grafting was still missing. This omission has now been rectified by Dr. Klasen.

This book is an expansion of a M.D. thesis, written at the State University of Groningen, The Netherlands, and was guided by Professor A. J. C. Huffstadt, plastic surgeon, and Professor D. de Moulin, medical historian. Professor T. Gibson kindly revised the manuscript and wrote the epilogue. But, as Goethe put it: "nur ein Teil der Kunst kann gelehrt werden, der Künstler macht das Ganze" ("only a part of the art can be taught, the artist makes the totality").

The author, Henk Klasen, is a remarkable man. As a general surgeon, he devotes all his interest and skills to traumatology and problems of physiology and pathophysiology in surgery. With such talents it is natural that he also works parttime as one of the coordinators of a modern burn unit.

Among his hobbies are love of antiques and old books.

This historical inclination has induced him to write the present book, in which he vividly describes the development of free skin grafting in its relevant theoretical and practical aspects. His elaborate study has resulted in an excellent reference book which at the same time provides enjoyable reading, once again demonstrating the value of history in understanding the present.

A. J. C. Huffstadt, M.D.
D. de Moulin, M.D.

Preface

A period of more than 100 years separates the first free skin graft from skin grafts as they are performed today. In this time, several aspects of skin grafting have evolved step by step.

This thesis presents an account of this evolution and discusses such aspects as indications, grafting methods, preparations, technical procedures, and the evaluation of results.

The data for this survey were obtained from the literature, comprising British, American, German, French, Scandinavian, Swiss, Austrian, Russian, and Dutch journals and books. Publications which could not be traced were not included.

The evolution of various aspects of skin grafting is discussed in chronological order. First, a survey is presented of attempts at skin grafting prior to Reverdin's invention. The chapter which discusses Reverdin's method of skin grafting illustrates the great influence of skin grafting on the treatment of wounds and ulcers.

A separate chapter is devoted to the importance of skin grafting in palpebral surgery. In this branch of surgery, skin grafting had an entirely separate development.

The next chapter outlines the importance of Thiersch and his influence on his contemporaries.

The evolution of various aspects of skin grafting in the 20th century is discussed in two chapters. One covers the period from about 1900 to 1930, while the other deals with the period from about 1930 to 1950. The periods are rather arbitrarily chosen. The year 1900 is convenient because at that time in general the interest in skin grafting had decreased, but during and after World War I the interest increased again. In the period of 1930–1950, World War II was a dominant factor. During the war and thereafter up to 1950, many new developments were published. In a few cases in which the year 1950 did not signify the end of some particular development, publications of a later date are also included.

The term "skin grafting" will be frequently used. Skin grafting will be defined as "transfer of skin from one site of the body to another, with complete interruption of the blood supply".

Occasionally, the pleonasm "free skin graft" will be used in order to avoid confusion with (pedicled) flap. Flaps are sometimes incorrectly referred to as "grafts" (Rogers 1959). In flaps, however, the blood supply is not interrupted completely.

We define "split-skin grafts" as grafts which consist of epidermis and part of the corium, whereas "full-thickness grafts" comprise the epidermis and the entire corium together.

For the reader's convenience, efforts have been made to ensure optimal uniformity of terminology. In some instances, terms are used which differ from those used by the authors in their original publications.

The term "autografting" is used when the donor is the same individual as the recipient.

Since this is a historical survey, it is regarded as justifiable to use the "old-fashioned" terms "homografting" and "heterografting" rather than the currently more widely employed terms "allografting" and "xenografting". Homografting (allografting) is the transfer of a graft from one individual to another individual of the same species. Heterografting (xenografting) is the transfer of a graft from one individual to another of a different species.

H. J. Klasen

Table of Contents

Chapter 1
Experiences With and Views on Skin Grafting Prior to Reverdin's Invention (1869)

Nearly all historical reviews on skin grafting refer to India, where the technique is believed to have been used for centuries; by way of illustration, Dutrochet's article in the French *Gazette de Santé* (Dutrochet 1817) is then mentioned. The widely quoted article was actually a letter to the editor in which Dutrochet, a physician, recounted the experiences of his brother-in-law. The latter, a high-ranking army officer in India, had described the following events to Dutrochet:

> An officer serving under the brother-in-law had punished one of his subordinates by having the man's nose cut off. The man then sought out Indians who were known for their ability to reconstruct a nose by surgery, and requested them to perform this operation on him.

Next, Dutrochet described the operation which the Indians were believed to have performed on this man:

> Because the defect was already showing cicatrization, the wound edges were freshened. One of the man's buttocks, which was to be the donor site, was beaten with an old shoe until a substantial swelling was achieved. From this swollen area, a triangular piece of skin, with subcutaneous fat, was then cut and placed on the defect. It was fixed in position with adhesive plaster. The graft healed, and the man continued to serve in the brother-in-law's command.

While this case history is not entirely impossible, the last line in the second case history cannot be true:

> A man had been caught looting, and one of his ears was cut off by way of punishment. The man wanted a new ear, but his own ear had been thrown away and could not be found. The ear of a pariah was therefore bought, cut off and used to replace the ear of the punished man. The grafting was successful . . .

At the end of his letter Dutrochet mentioned that he himself had made several attempts at grafting on animals, but that none had been successful. He assumed that this was due to the fact that the grafts had not been prepared (by beating).

This article has some incredible passages, which cast doubt on its veracity. The reliability of the article was indeed soon considered debatable. Zeis (1863) qualified the experiences recounted in the article as fables (the fact that he could react to the article 46 years after its publication illustrates that the medical literature of that time did not become outdated as quickly as in our time). He pointed out that this had been a single publication, and that nothing had since been heard about skin grafting in India. Marchand (1901) called Dutrochet's story a fantasy which mixed the operation of the pedicled flap with legend. Nevertheless the article attracted much attention and was translated in several foreign medical journals. Sometimes only a part of the article was published (Dittmer 1817; Villeneuve 1817). Gibson (1963) discovered that the English translation did not come from the *Gazette de Santé* of 1817, but from a version published by Blandin (1836). Unfortunately, Blandin had mentioned only the first of the two case histories of the original article and ignored the case history of the ear transplantation.

Brock (1952) described how Sir Astley Cooper (1768–1841) in London had successfully performed a human skin graft in 1817. Cooper had already shown his particular interest in transplantations by several experiments. The description of this operation was recorded in a rough notebook Cooper kept for notes on museum specimens, surgical procedures and other accounts. The abstract was written by an unknown person.

> Hartfield was a young man admitted into Guys Hospital (Cornelius Ward) on April 9th 1817, with a diseased thumb which Mr. Cooper, now Sir Astley, amputated between the phalanges on the 18th of July. He then cut off a healthy piece of integument from the amputated part and applied it to the face of the stump where he secured it by means of adhesive slips.
>
> *1st week to July 25th,* union seems to have taken place.
>
> *2nd week to August 1st,* Mr. Cooper proved the vascularity of the newly attached portion by pricking it very slightly with a point of a lancet, which produced fluid blood as readily as from any other part of the joint. Sensibility has not returned.
>
> *3rd week from operation.* In the course of this week sensation has returned in the end of the stump.
>
> *September 23rd,* the stump appeared quite well. [1]

A year later, in 1818 and 1819, three newly graduated Dutch physicians (Tilanus, Broers and De Fremery) made a hiking tour to various European university cities. In the course of this tour they visited the university of Marburg in Germany, and made the acquaintance of Bünger, professor of anatomy and surgery. Bünger received them cordially and gave them an account of several case histories, including one which involved a successful skin graft. One of the visitors (Tilanus) recorded Bünger's observations about this operation in his diary (Deelman 1925).

It was not until three years later that a report on this skin graft was published in the *Journal der Chirurgie und Augen-Heilkunde* (Bünger 1822) (Fig. 1), at the explicit invitation of one of the editors of the journal (Gräfe 1821).

Bünger described in detail why he had not used a pedicled flap, as some surgeons were already doing at that time. The anatomical situation had more or less forced him to resort to a free skin graft. Bünger and an assistant inspected the wound on the third day after grafting, in the presence of several of the patient's relatives. In a moving account of what he and his assistant felt when they saw that the graft was taking, Bünger wrote:

> Wir Aertze sahen uns nur starr an, und trauten erst unsern Augen nicht, indem wir den Tags zuvor kreideweissen Lappen, der wenigstens anderthalb Stunden dem Lebenseinflusse vom übrigen Körper entzogen gewesen war, jetzt in der Form einer Nase an dem beträchtlichsten Teile seiner Oberfläche rein scharlachroth glänzend und aufgedunsen erblickten ... [2]

---

1 This case history has also been mentioned by Zimmerman and Veith (1961) and by Balch and Marzoni (1977).

2 We doctors looked at each other in silence and did not believe our eyes when we saw that a graft which the day before had been chalk-white and had been deprived of the vital forces from the remainder of the body for at least 90 minutes, now had become a nose which for the most part had a pure scarlet colour and looked glossy and swollen ...

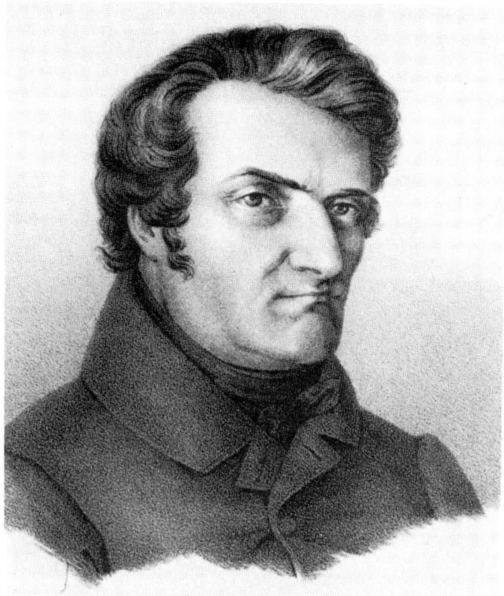

Fig. 1. Christian Heinrich Bünger (1782 – 1842), anatomist and surgeon in Marburg, Germany, who performed the first, well documented full thickness skin grafting in 1817

Bünger's attempt had been inspired by Dutrochet's report in the *Gazette de Santé*. Although he had had his doubts about the method, he thought an attempt would do little harm to the patient.

Transplantation was performed to replace the nose of a woman of 33 years old. Except that the woman had been very pretty before her nose was destroyed by a destructive process and that she had already visited many doctors, Bünger gave no information about the patient or her illness.

He did not use a buttock as donor site, as mentioned in Dutrochet's story, because this would inconvenience the patient and impede sitting and lying. Another argument was that wound toilet and the changing of dressings would be difficult. He therefore selected the venterolateral aspect of the upper thigh as donor site. In accordance with the Indian example, this area was beaten with a leather belt until the skin looked red and swollen. A piece of skin measuring 10×7.5 cm was then excised, with half of the thickness of the layer of subcutaneous fat attached. The graft was then trimmed to the desired shape and used to "replace" the malformed nose. The graft was fixed to the freshened wound surface by means of sutures. The dressing, consisting of a layer of cotton wool, was fixed in position with adhesive plaster.

The graft still looked dead-white on the second postoperative day, but one day later it had assumed a reddish colour, with the exception of the lower edge which was blue. As Bünger had feared, this edge became necrotic and it had to be excised on the ninth postoperative day.

Five weeks after the operation, all skin defects had healed. The layer of dry, dead epidermis had been shed much earlier. After healing, the reconstructed nose was growing the same kind of hairs as the donor site. One year after the operation the grafted skin still differed in colour from the rest of the face.

Not long after Bünger's description Dieffenbach (1824 a) a celebrated German surgeon, and one of the founders of plastic surgery in Germany, published his report on a skin graft that he had performed largely as an experiment.

This was part of the treatment of a 40-year-old woman suffering from sensory disorders and reduced muscular strength in the left half of the body. The physicians in charge believed that application of exogenous stimuli to the anaesthetic half of the body would have a beneficial effect on the disease process. Dieffenbach assumed that this could best be achieved by a kind of "exchange" skin graft. Prior to grafting, the skin on the flexor side of the forearm was stimulated by rubbing with alcohol, Dieffenbach apparently being influenced in this regard by Dutrochet's publication. A piece of skin the size of a thaler (diameter: 35 mm) was cut from this area 24 h later. The thickness of the graft was not specified. A skin fragment of the same dimensions was excised from the extensor side of the forearm, without previously stimulating the area. The portions of skin were exchanged and placed in the fresh wounds. They were held in position by means of adhesive plaster. The wounds were inspected after six days. The graft placed on the flexor side of the forearm "floated in pus"; the epidermis was still attached to it. The "prepared" graft placed on the extensor side of the forearm looked quite different. The epidermis had become detached, half of the graft had become putrified, but the remainder was attached to the underlying structures and was surrounded by granulation tissue. Unfortunately, this fragment was inadvertently pulled loose from the underlying structures when the dressing was changed, whereupon both graft and wound began to bleed. According to Dieffenbach, the bleeding proved that the circulation had meanwhile been restored. Both skin defects subsequently healed within a few days. It was in fact even claimed that there was no scar.

Apart from this clinical experiment, Dieffenbach (1824 b, 1830) performed many experiments in an effort to establish the feasibility of skin grafting in birds, rabbits, cats and dogs. Not only was skin grafted from one bird to another but also from mammals to birds. All these attempts failed because the grafts became desiccated. Dieffenbach suspected that this was due to the high body temperature of the birds. In another experiment, a piglet's skin was grafted on a pigeon. The graft dried out, but the hairs in the grafted skin were reported as having resumed growing after 8 days. The test animal was sacrificed 10 days after the operation. The graft was found to be attached to the wound floor, but was not vascularized. Other experiments in rabbits and dogs likewise failed.

In one rabbit, however, the tip of the nose was successfully reattached. In one series of experiments, a piece of skin with a diameter of 1 cm was excised from rabbit ears, and reapplied to the area after haemostasis. Although the experiment was repeated as often as 50 times, only three rabbits showed reattachment of the skin. In these experiments, too, the vitality of the grafts was "stimulated" by rubbing and beating.

Attempts to graft skin at other sites, e.g. the back or the head in rabbits, also failed. In all cases the top layer of the graft, including the hair roots, was shed, where-upon epithelialization of the intact layer of the graft occurred.

Other attempts made by Dieffenbach to graft human skin were all failures. He made these attempts in patients in whom tumours had been extirpated. The skin which had covered the tumours was used to cover the defects. In none of these patients did the autografts take. Yet Dieffenbach was convinced that well-vascularized skin should be suitable for grafting. He expected that scrotal skin had the best characteristics for this purpose – an assumption based on the fact that, after excision, scrotal skin changed its size and shape. This skin, therefore, "had to be" still vital.

Dieffenbach's experiments were resumed in the same thorough way by Hanff of Berlin in 1870 (Hanff 1870). He was unaware of the successful skin graft performed by Reverdin in 1869. Hanff performed his experiments not to prove that tissues from certain parts of the body could grow at other sites (he considered this a proven fact), but to study the healing process. Grafting experiments were done on homoiothermic and poikilothermic animal species. The grafts consisted of skin, subcutaneous fat and fascia or muscle tissue. Hanff found that skin could be transplanted without difficulty from one frog to another. He did report, however, that bleeding occurred beneath the grafts 9–14 days after the operation, although the grafts had initially shown adequate attachment.

By that time the recipient frogs gave an impression of lassitude. Microscopic examination after sacrificing the animals revealed that the grafts had become attached to a thickened, highly cellularized fascia layer.

Hanff considered the frog the most suitable test animal for skin grafting because grafts could be easily obtained, and the subcutaneous fascia of the frog provided a good underlying structure for grafting. Attempts to graft frog skin onto wounds covered with granulation tissue failed.

Hanff concluded from his frog experiments that the graft had to be larger than the defect to be covered; that after 2–3 days the epidermis, with the Malpighian layer, detached itself from the rest of the graft, and that grafts were nourished via the floor of the wound.

Hanff's experiments on poikilothermic species consisted of autografting, homografting and heterografting in dogs and rats. The grafts consisted of skin together with a layer of subcutis. After haemostasis, the grafts were applied without any tension and sutured. Hanff observed that the grafts initially attached themselves, but became detached after 9–12 days. In his evaluation of results he made no distinction between autografts, homografts and heterografts. None of these grafts healed completely; partial healing was observed in three cases (he did not specify whether these were autografts).

Hanff maintained that graft healing was a stepwise process. The superficial graft parts furthest from the nourishing wound bed ran the gravest risk of becoming necrotic. The grafting result depended on the speed of revascularization and the progressive degeneration of the graft. A few hours after operation the graft was already attached to the wound bed. This phenomenon deeply impressed Hanff, and was emphatically mentioned several times. After 24 hours, union between graft and wound floor should have been established – as manifested by swelling of the grafts. Although he considered this a favourable omen, it did not imply that healing would in fact occur. Further healing was effected in that the graft was incorporated in the vascular system, but this took some more time. During this period the graft was prevented from degenerating by an "inflammatory plastic" (entzündlich-plastisch) process.

This process was nothing but the inflammatory reaction which in his opinion was always associated with grafting. White blood corpuscles were already present in the wound 4–6 hours after infliction.

According to Hanff, these white blood corpuscles were converted to connective tissue cells after 48 hours. The "plastic" reaction then ceased, and granulation tissue was formed, which then enclosed the graft. Once the granulation tissue had interposed itself between grafted tissue and wound floor, Hanff believed, the relation between floor and graft was established. Direct adhesion of graft to wound floor, he maintained, did not prevent the inflammatory reaction but did prevent the suppuration which occurred in other wounds. The white corpuscles, Hanff assumed, probably played a role in suppuration. He expected that white corpuscles might also turn into tissue cells. The zone in which suppuration occurred formed the boundary between the vital and the dead graft tissue. Hanff believed that, via the blood vessels, the white corpuscles entered the exudate between wound floor and transplant, and then infiltrated the graft; subsequently, the blood vessels supplying the graft were formed. He therefore assumed an unmistakable relation between the presence of leucocytes in the graft and the restoration of the circulation. Moreover, he was convinced that granulation tissue and the "plastic, infiltrative" reaction in the graft were produced by the same process. Graft healing was therefore to be expected up to the layer in which these reactions occurred, but the more superficial layers would degenerate. Once the degenerated tissue was shed, epidermis (he probably meant epithelium) was formed from the wound edges; and this covered the intact part of the graft.

Hanff concluded that grafts degenerated unless early vascularization developed. Since skin consisted largely of connective tissue, it was more resistant than most other tissues and therefore the most suitable for grafting. Hanff considered the loss of "epidermis" in skin grafting to be of secondary importance, and he maintained that the significance of the serous transudation should not be underrated. In his opinion, attempts to stimulate the vitality of the graft by provoking an inflammatory reaction (by alcohol rubbing or beating, according to the ancient Indian rules) were of little value.

The work of Hanff did not attract much attention because of the earlier invention of Reverdin. However it should be appreciated that Hanff was the first to describe extensive microscopic studies in this field, which became possible through the development of histological colouring techniques, good microtomes and improvements to the microscope.

References

Balch CM, Marzoni FA (1977) Skin transplantation during the pre-Reverdin era, 1804–1869. Surg Gynecol Obstet 144:766

Blandin PF (1836) De l'autoplastie. Urtubie, Paris

Brock RC (1952) The life and work of Astley Cooper. Livingstone, Edinburgh, p 47

Bünger CH (1822) Gelungener Versuch einer Nasenbildung aus einem völlig getrennten Hautstück aus dem Beine. J Chir Augen-Heilk 4:569

Deelman HT (1925) Surgery: a hundred years ago. Bles, London
Dieffenbach JF (1824 a) Ueberpflanzung völlig getrennter Hautstücke bei einer Frau, und Wiederanheilung einer grössen Theils abgehauenen Wange. J Chir Augen-Heilk 6:482
Dieffenbach JF (1824 b) Transplantationsversuche bei Thieren. J Chir Augen-Heilk 6:122
Dieffenbach JF (1830) Chirurgische Erfahrungen, besonders über die Wiederherstellung zerstörter Theile des menschlichen Körpers. Enslin, Berlin
Dittmer (1817) Kurze Nachrichten und Auszüge: Neue und noch bequemere Methode Nasen zu restauriren. J practischen Heilkunde 94:106
Dutrochet H (1817) Gaz Santé 35:91 (Translations in McDowell F (1977) The source book of plastic surgery. Williams & Wilkins, Baltimore, p 105 and Plast Reconstr Surg 1969, 44:288)
Gibson T (1963) Flagellation and free grafting. Br J Plast Surg 13:195
Gräfe CF (1821) Neue Beiträge zur Kunst, Theile des Angesichts organisch zu ersetzen. J Chir Augen-Heilk 2:1
Hanff W (1870) Ueber Wiederanheilung vollständig vom Körper getrennter Hautstücke. Inaugural thesis, Lange, Berlin Friedrich-Wilhelms-Universität (Berlin)
Marchand F (1901) Der Process der Wundheilung. Enke, Stuttgart
Villeneuve ACL (1817) Précis des Journaux. J Med Chir Pharm 39:91
Zeis E (1863) Die Literatur und Geschichte der plastischen Chirurgie. Engelmann, Leipzig
Zimmerman LM, Veith I (1961) Great ideas in the history of surgery. Williams & Wilkins, Baltimore, p 400

Chapter 2
Skin Grafting by the Reverdin Method and Subsequent Developments

A. The Skin Grafts of Jaques-Louis Reverdin

Jaques-Louis Reverdin (Fig. 2) was born in Geneva, where he also spent his youth. In 1862 he went to Paris for his medical training, and in 1869 he started work as a resident under Felix Guyon [1] at the Hôpital Necker. On 8th December 1869, Reverdin addressed a meeting of the Société Impériale de Chirurgie de Paris with a paper entitled "Greffe épidermique". In the introduction to his paper

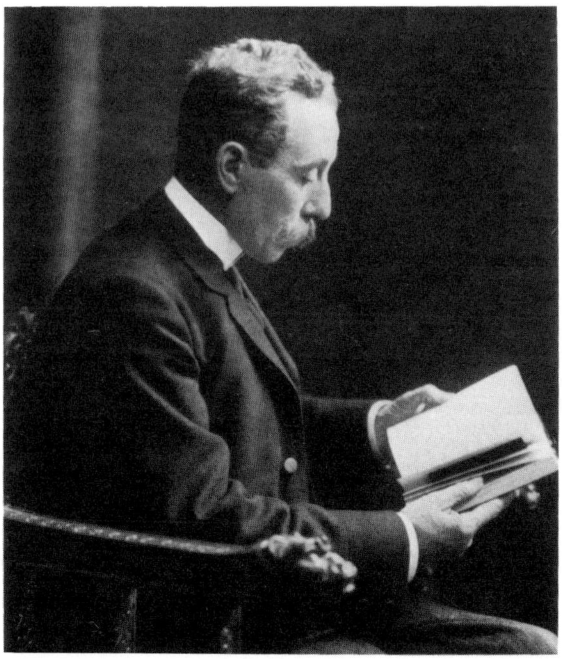

Fig. 2. Jaques-Louis Reverdin (1842 – 1929), who developed a practicable method of skin grafting (Reverdin 1971)

1 Professor in surgical pathology and one of the founders of modern urology.

he emphasized that he wanted to speak about wound healing by second intention. As a resident in surgery he had been involved in the treatment of a 35-year-old man, who had sustained an injury of the forearm with total detachment of the skin. Thirty-nine days after the accident, the skin defect was covered with fresh granulation tissue. When Reverdin examined the wound, he remembered that islands with epithelium sometimes formed in the centre of the granulation tissue in patients with burns. [2] These islands significantly accelerated healing. He therefore wondered whether the duration of healing in this patient might be reduced by placing fragments of epidermis in the wound. Through this original thinking a new principle was introduced by which Reverdin trod a different path from Bünger and Dieffenbach.

From the patient's other arm he cut two small, thin skin fragments: one had a surface area of about 1 mm^2, and the other was even smaller. These fragments were placed close together on the granulation tissue in the centre of the wound, and pressed firmly in position. A dressing with diachylon ointment was applied to secure the skin fragments. When the wound was examined the next day, the fragments were still in position although the wound surface showed abundant suppuration. Six days after the operation the skin fragments seemed to have increased in size, and a layer of epidermis had formed around them. These annular zones became so wide, within 14 days, that the two islands grew together. Reverdin unfortunately failed to specify the original distance between the two skin fragments. He read a paper on this subject 15 days after the operation. His teacher Guyon

---

2 Reverdin referred to Billroth, who in 1866 had described the process of wound healing in *Handbuch der Allgemeinen und speciellen Chirurgie* (Billroth 1866). In order to gain some insight into the theories on wound healing in Reverdin's time it seems useful to outline some of the observations on wound healing that were propounded by Billroth:

A thick yellow fluid appeared on the wound floor three days after infliction of the wound. Dead tissue fragments disappeared from the wound surface which itself became smoother and redder. At that time small nodules were visible with a magnifying glass. After 4–6 days the nodules had become large enough to give the wound surface a granular appearance. The pus became thicker. Billroth mentioned this beneficial or "laudable" pus. He regarded pus as liquefied inflammatory or granulation tissue. Even after publication of the monograph of Koch (1878) "Untersuchungen über die Aetiologie der Wundinfektionskrankheiten" which established the fact that specific bacteria were responsible for infection of surgical wounds, Billroth stuck to his theories (Billroth 1879).

The nodules of the granulation tissue gradually increased in size and finally aggregated so that no separate individual nodules were distinguishable any more. The granulation tissue became more and more elevated, usually to the level of the adjacent skin, sometimes even higher.

Cicatrization also began in the course of this process, and the wound surface contracted. The pus production diminished in the zone of transition between skin and granulation tissue. This zone assumed a redder colour. It gradually moved towards the centre of the wound and was followed by a light-blue-to-white zone of epithelium which merged into normal epidermis. The cicatrix moved over a distance of 1–2 mm every day. The young cicatricial tissue had a red colour, was firm to touch and adherent to the underlying structures.

Billroth also noticed that cicatrization sometimes started from islands in the centre of the granulation tissue. In his opinion this was only possible if a fragment of skin with its Malpighian layer had remained intact, as it sometimes was in burns. However thin the Malpighian layer was, epidermis always formed again. He was convinced however that a cicatricial island could never develop spontaneously in a wound.

undoubtedly played a role in this respect. He had immediately understood the importance of this development, and wanted Reverdin to go on record in speech and writing as soon as possible. One day after reading his paper, on 9th December 1869, Reverdin wrote a letter to his parents in Geneva to inform them of what he described as his small invention, and to explain why this had been publicized so hastily:

> . . . I have recently carried out a small experiment which appeared to me to be of some theoretical, and perhaps also of some practical importance. Since the experiment was new and entirely my own, my chief, Mr. Guyon, told me to report it to the Société de Chirurgie, and arranged for me to speak last Wednesday. Even though I had only one case to report, I took the opportunity, if only to fix the date of my small invention, because the non-residents and my students had begun to talk about it, so that anyone could have claimed it. (Reverdin 1971)

The meeting did not respond too enthusiastically to Reverdin's report. Le Fort and Blot, well-known doctors, for example, remarked that the donor sites might well become portals of entry for other disease processes, such as erysipelas.

Despite the reluctant response of the meeting, the free skin graft as invented by Reverdin seems to have been widely used in France, and especially in Paris, although the French literature on this subject is scanty (Reverdin 1872; H. Reverdin 1971). It was not until months later that the invention became known in other countries. One of the reasons was that Paris was isolated from the rest of the world owing to the Franco-Prussian War of 1870–1871.

This isolation precluded contacts with medical colleagues elsewhere. The first country to use the free skin grafts of Reverdin on large scale was Great Britain.

Pollock, a surgeon at St. George's Hospital, and consulting surgeon at the Hospital for Sick Children in Great Ormond Street, played an important role in this context. In May 1870 he heard from a former pupil, Bowles, who had just returned from France, that Reverdin in Paris could accelerate the healing of large wound surfaces with the aid of free skin grafts. Pollock then started to use the method, and with great success, as will be discussed later. His name was subsequently mentioned frequently in British medical journals. (Editorial 1870 a, b, c) and many other British surgeons started to make use of free skin grafts. From Great Britain, the free skin graft was introduced in several other countries (e.g. Germany, Austria, America, Russia and Scandinavia) by surgeons who had watched the procedure in England. In the Netherlands transplantation was little used.

It was however never doubted that the honour of the invention was Reverdin's. Pollock and Reverdin expressed considerable mutual respect and appreciation in their publications. In November 1870, Pollock expressed in the *Lancet* his disappointment at being unable to contact Reverdin in any way. He wrote that the "state of Paris" had forbidden any contact (Pollock 1870 d).

When Reverdin had finished his training in Paris, in 1872, he made a tour of Europe before establishing himself as a surgeon in Geneva. In the course of this tour he also visited London, where he met Pollock several times. He even wrote to his parents from England that Pollock's son was to come and work with him in Geneva (Reverdin 1971).

In 1872, Reverdin published an article describing the state of affairs of free skin grafting which will be discussed in the next section.

The *Académie de Paris* awarded this publication the *Prix Amussat,* thus expressing French recognition of Reverdin's invention; of course Pollock was mentioned several times in this publication. It is remarkable that Reverdin, who from 1869 to 1872 published four articles on skin grafting, did not write a single paper on the subject after 1872.

Reverdin's Technique of Skin Grafting

The way in which Reverdin applied the free skin graft was probably the best solution conceivable at the time of its introduction. The operation was simple and it has to be admitted that Reverdin cared neither for antisepsis nor anaesthesia. Antisepsis was already known (Lister 1827–1912 had reported on antiseptic wound management in 1867), although it was by no means already generally practised. Asepsis was still an unknown concept. Another aid without which skin grafting is hardly feasible today – anaesthesia – was used only sparingly in Reverdin's day. [3]

This reluctance to use anaesthesia was probably due to the complications associated with it. Local anaesthesia with the aid of cocaine was still unknown until Koller (1857–1944) introduced it in 1884 to anaesthetize the cornea.

The technique which Reverdin used was hardly painful because the skin fragments taken were minute, so there seemed to be no need for anaesthesia. The procedure was simple and quick. Although it is difficult to establish this with certainty, we may assume that many skin grafts were performed in the patients' homes, because at that time it was quite normal to perform operations at home, especially for the well-to-do. Only in a few case reports is this mentioned by the authors themselves (Bellamy 1870; Clemens 1875; Coombs 1876).

Indication for a Reverdin Skin Graft

General Indications

When after Reverdin's first report it became known that healing by second intention could be accelerated with the aid of skin grafts, they were applied to virtually all skin defects. This caused many disappointments. Probably this was one of the reasons why the method, after its initial sudden rise, lost its popularity fairly quickly in subsequent years.

After his first attempt, Reverdin asked himself in which patients the grafts might be effectively used, and what the future value of the method might be. A few years later (1872), he himself answered these questions. He reached the conclusion that skin grafts could be used to reduce the duration of healing of therapy-resistant skin defects and skin defects in which healing was slow and laborious. He held that free skin grafting ensured a strong, flexible scar which was less readily disrupted than a scar obtained without grafting. He also suggested that contraction of tissues around the wound could be prevented by skin grafting (Fig. 3).

---

3 The use of ether as an anaesthetic had been introduced by Long in 1842 and Morton in 1846. In 1844, Wells had described a mixture of nitrous oxide and oxygen as a useful aid, and Simpson had introduced chloroform in 1847.

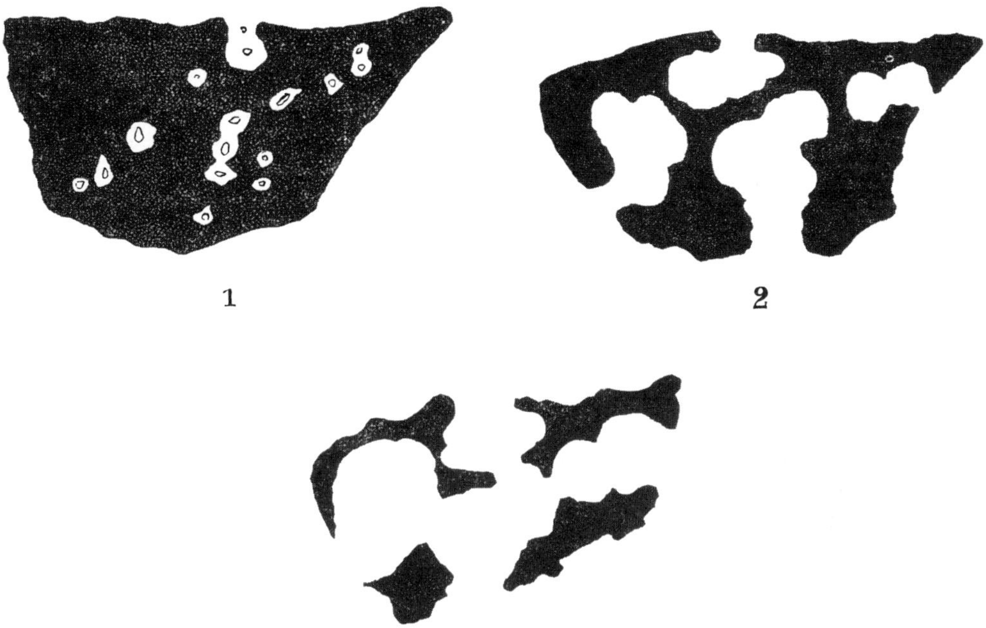

Fig. 3. Illustrations in an article of Reverdin (1872). The results of skin grafting are shown. Epithelium spreads from the grafts and the wound edges. The epithelial islands confluate until the whole surface ist epithelialized

In his opinion, skin grafting would be of value in particular in the management of large burns, large sores, periarticular wounds (to prevent ankylosis) and conical skin defects caused by amputation. Although the first patient on whom Reverdin used a skin graft had lost skin in an accident with a machine, Reverdin believed that skin grafting might be of particular value in the management of burns; and when he had occasion to treat a patient with burns one month after his first attempt, he immediately took his chance.

... In 1867 a 36-year-old man burned his leg against a stove. The burn had healed almost entirely six months later, but a skin defect persisted. Because the defect had increased in size again, the patient was treated as an in-patient at the Hôpital Necker in October 1869.

Careful, consistent treatment by conservative measures failed to cause healing of the defect. There remained an ulcer measuring 13 × 7 cm, the floor of which showed little inclination to granulate. Guyon proposed that Reverdin apply skin fragments from an amputated leg to the ulcer, but the patient refused to receive skin from somebody else. On 13th January 1870, a few skin fragments from the patient himself were applied to the scanty granulations in the ulcer. (The patient evidently did not object to this!) One graft took and became a "cicatricial island". The appearance of the ulcer floor improved, and new skin grafts were subsequently implanted at regular intervals. In March 1870 the defect was not yet entirely closed, and new skin fragments from other patients (including a negro) were applied to the ulcer.

We read that "complete healing of the ulcer was achieved in June 1870" (Reverdin 1872).

This case history is presented in such detail here, because Freshwater and Krizek (1971) concluded that Pollock had been the first surgeon to use skin grafts on a patient with burns. The above case history disproves this conclusion, for it was not until May 1870 that Pollock performed his first skin graft (Pollock 1870 a, b, c, d, 1871). The first patient whom Pollock treated was an 8-year-old girl who had sustained burns of the leg in 1868. Two years after this accident she still showed a skin defect, and Pollock applied his first skin grafts to this defect in May 1870. Several other grafts followed, and the defect was completely healed six months after the first operation. This announcement by Pollock elicited an editorial note in the *Lancet* only three months after the operation, stating that the results of skin grafting looked promising, and that skin grafts might well be a new asset in the treatment of patients with large burns; not only might they reduce the duration of illness but they might also prevent the frequently resulting deformities (Editorial 1870 a, b). At first this assumption was shared by almost everyone. The great value of skin grafts in the management of burns was recognized by virtually all surgeons (Dobson 1870 a, b, c; Steele 1870; Chisolm 1871; Ranke 1871; Forster 1872; Bryant 1872). They all regarded the prevention of deformities as one of the principal indications for skin grafting. Skin grafts were recommended also for patients with skin defects due to other injuries (Wurfbain 1871; Jacenko 1871 b; Donnelly 1872; Larrey 1872). Trueheart (1871) also advised grafting for skin defects caused by gun shot wounds. Grafting was emphatically recommended for patients who had lost skin from the scalp in accidents with machines, because these patients otherwise died from complications. Scalping wounds caused enormous defects. Sometimes it took years before the wounds were healed (Netolitzky 1871; Bartlett 1872; Burdel 1875; Reverdin 1876; Abbe 1878; Finnell 1878; Cowell 1879; Brown 1879; Bradley 1881; Gussenbauer 1883).

It is worthy of note that skin grafts continued to be used for such patients even when grafting had become less popular owing to disappointing results.

Skin grafts were also applied to surgical skin defects e.g. in patients treated by amputation of a limb (an operation which often left a conical skin defect that failed to heal). On such patients Jacenko (1871 b) and Reverdin (1872), among others, performed skin grafts. Skin grafting was also advised for skin defects resulting from non-specific or specific inflammatory processes (Steele 1870; Storch 1871; Jacenko 1871 b; Rodriguez 1871). Heiberg and Schultz (1871) may be specially mentioned in this respect. They worked at a Berlin military hospital where soldiers with erysipelas were treated. In over 50 patients, skin defects were treated with skin grafts. (Erysipelas was one of the horrors of the 19th century.)

Most publications on skin grafting concerned the treatment of patients with ulcers of the lower leg (Kempe 1870; Lamm 1870; Couper 1870; Lawson 1870 a, b, 1871; Croft 1870; Mesterton 1871; Morales 1871; Bryant 1871; Kappeler 1871; Hofmokl 1871; Donnelly 1872); in most cases the cause of the ulcers was not mentioned. It is not surprising that skin grafts were so frequently used particularly in these cases. Ulcers of the leg were quite common, and no method had so far succeeded in producing permanent healing. Most efforts to treat ulcers of the leg failed and ended in the most radical solution: amputation.

Other, less frequently mentioned indications for skin grafting were decubitus ulcers (Kappeler 1871) and granulating skin defects following excision of tumours, e.g. tumours of the breast (Heath 1870). Anderson (1871) summarized the indications for skin grafting. He regarded it as a means to achieve rapid cicatrization of any granulating surface, especially wounds which showed insufficient or no inclination to heal spontaneously. He also raised the question whether skin grafting might be preferable as well in granulating skin defects which did tend to heal spontaneously.

The grafts could then be used to reduce the duration of healing and prevent contraction of the tissues. With regard to the last-mentioned indication, Anderson (1871) expressed the views prevalent among British surgeons. In most other countries, skin grafts were hardly used for this purpose.

Looking for Indications in Reconstructive Surgery

It was soon understood that skin grafting might also be of importance in repairing skin defects resulting from excisions in cases in which other ways of supplying skin (e.g. pedicled flaps) were impracticable. This problem was especially encountered in patients with contractures after burns (Steele, 1870). Jacenko (1871 a) even assumed that free skin grafts might entirely replace pedicled flaps in future. On the other hand however, there were surgeons who considered skin grafts to be of no value in reconstructive surgery (Heiberg 1871 a; Bryant 1871, 1872).

In England too, attempts to use skin grafts in reconstructions were made within a few months of the introduction of skin grafting. Mason (1870 a) of the Westminster Hospital in London published an interesting report in the *Lancet* of August 1870:

> A young woman had sustained deep burns of the cervical region, which had healed with severe contractions. The chin and lower lip were pulled down as a result. The cicatricial tissue which caused these contractures was excised, and six to eight small skin grafts were applied to the fresh skin defect.

Later, Mason (1870 b) reported that the attempt had failed completely. He assumed that it had failed because the grafts had been insufficiently fixed in position. The site of the intervention precluded adequate immobilization. Even today, nobody will deny that reconstructions in the cervical region are among the most difficult ventures of plastic surgery, particularly in patients with burns. Steele (1870) made a similar attempt in a boy with dermatogenic contracture of the elbow resulting from burns: after excision of the cicatricial adhesions, the fresh wound surface was covered with a few square millimetres of skin graft. This operation likewise failed, according to Steele because the grafts had been applied to a fresh wound surface!

In other countries, too, attempts were made to use skin grafts in reconstructive surgery. Menzel (1872) described such a procedure, carried out by Billroth. He attempted to reconstruct a nose with the aid of skin grafts. He, too, applied the grafts to the fresh wound surface. His attempt failed, and this failure was again ascribed to the fresh wound surface. Later (1879), Billroth himself reported that he used skin flaps to repair the skin defects resulting from excision of cicatricial tissue in patients with contractures. Unfortunately, he presented no further details on the results.

In another patient, who had likewise developed severe contractures in the cervical region after burns, Pollock (1871) excised the cicatricial tissue, waited seven days, and then applied skin grafts to the granulation tissue. This attempt also failed. In September 1870 Arnott, of the Middlesex Hospital in London, attempted another corrective procedure which poses grave problems even today:

A pretty girl had sustained a burn of the cervical region five months previously. The burn had healed with keloid formation (or so it was at least described by Arnott). The ugly scar inconvenienced the patient. Arnott excised the elevated tissue and, two weeks later covered the resulting skin defect, of unknown size, with two small (pea-sized) skin grafts. Two additional grafts were applied "some time later". Three weeks after the first graft the wound had healed almost entirely, with a soft scar in which not a trace of swelling could be detected, according to Arnott. The "result" of the intervention was published four weeks after the first operation. No data on long-term healing can be found.

In general in the medical literature of the 19th century little attention was paid to long-term results.

A later complication of burns and its treatment was described by Poncet (1871), one of Ollier's pupils. He described how Ollier performed a skin graft on a defect resulting from excision of a tumour. (Ollier, professor of surgery at Lyon, was one of the best-known French surgeons.) The ulcerating tumour had developed in the scar of burns, which the patient had sustained 25 years before. The tumour was diagnosed as "epithelioma". Some time after excision of the tumour, skin grafts were applied to the skin defect in two sessions. Complete healing was achieved.

Ollier himself (1872 a, b) also reported on the good results he had obtained in reconstruction of syndactyly. He separated the fingers and used skin grafts to repair the resulting defects. He did not specify in his publications after what interval he applied the grafts, but Poncet wrote that this was always done after granulation tissue had developed. Ollier stressed that the concept of skin grafting encompassed more than the application of epithelial centres from which epithelialization might take place. He maintained that secondary epithelialization had to be prevented as far as possible, and that defects should entirely be covered with grafts which consisted of the full thickness of skin. His objective was to achieve a scar which had the same features as the adjacent normal skin; he accepted the absence of glandular structures in the grafting area as inevitable, although he realized that the quality of the scar was less good as a result.

A quite different use of skin grafts was described by Beigel (1872), a German and a former professor at the Charing Cross Hospital in London.

In two women with vaginal ulcers, he applied skin grafts to the floor of the ulcers, which subsequently healed. One year later there were still no indications of a relapse. Beigel failed to specify the aetiology of the ulcers.

One of the most important applications of skin grafts in reconstructive surgery – in the reconstruction of eyelids – will not be discussed here. A separate chapter is devoted to this subject because skin grafts in palpebral surgery went through a different evolution and attained a separate position.

Criteria Applied to the Wound

Reverdin (1869) performed his first skin graft on a granulating wound, and, afterwards, virtually all authors regarded the presence of granulation tissue as a prerequisite for a successful operation. Despite several unsuccessful attempts to apply skin grafts to a fresh wound surface, several surgeons remained convinced that this should be feasible as well. Anderson (1871), for example, wrote: "There is little doubt that the grafts could be made to take root on a freshly exposed surface." In the same year, this statement was corroborated by the German undergraduate Knie (1871). In an experiment on cats, Knie succeeded in having skin grafts take on a fresh wound surface. Although in subsequent years skin grafting on a fresh wound surface became firmly established in palpebral surgery, general surgeons continued to prefer grafting on granulating wound surfaces. Perhaps the technique and the vascularization of the wounds to which the grafts were applied played a role in this respect, although it is not mentioned in the literature. It was not until 1886 that Thiersch, to whom we will return later, proposed a different approach for grafting on fresh wound surfaces.

He had already made the same suggestion in 1874, but at that time had added that his experience was still insufficient to convince him completely of the advantages of this change of policy. After Thiersch's publication of 1874, Schede (1881) was virtually the only one to report on successful grafts on fresh wound surfaces. (Schede, of Hamburg, was distinguished in the field of general as well as in ophthalmic surgery.)

Not every granulation tissue was regarded as suitable; it had to be of good quality, that is: of firm consistency and fresh red appearance. In assessing the suitability of wounds for grafting, the wound edges were also considered. If they showed epithelialization or at least the inclination to epithelialize, the wound was accepted as suitable (Steele 1870; Reverdin 1872). The patient's general condition was a controversial point in considering the feasibility of grafting. Some surgeons regarded a good general condition as an absolute prerequisite (Pollock 1870 b, 1871; Wurfbain 1871; Bryant 1872), but others maintained that large wound surfaces influenced the general condition unfavourably, and that consequently grafting should not be postponed (Lindenbaum 1871).

Skin Grafting Technique

Preparation of the Wound

The literature gives no abundance of information on how the wounds were prepared. Several surgeons advised that irritants such as carbolic acid (phenol) be avoided during the last few days preceding grafting (Macleod 1871 b; Reverdin 1872). When the wounds showed little tendency to granulate, some surgeons tried to stimulate this with the aid of lint (Heiberg and Schulz 1871).

Silver nitrate (lunar caustic) was used to reduce excessive granulation. Prior to grafting, the wounds were as a rule intensively cleansed with water in order to remove "pus corpuscles" (Wood 1871; Kappeler 1871), and sometimes the wound was dried with swabs (Lindh 1872). Some surgeons brushed the granulation tissue until some slight bleeding occurred, and grafted when the bleeding ceased (Heiberg and Schulz 1871). Lochner (1872) scraped the granulations with a knife until he obtained a reddish surface.

Technique of Obtaining Grafts

In the 1870s and early 1880s, skin grafting was a simple, brief procedure. The wound surface received hardly any specific preparation. The grafts were obtained with simple, everyday instruments. The surgeons performed the operation with bare hands, without any antiseptic precaution.

Reverdin presented a detailed description of the way in which he excised the skin fragment to be used for grafting. As a donor site he usually selected the medial aspect of the leg at the level of the tibia. The skin was first shaven, lest hairs on the graft should stick to the dressing and cause accidental removal of the graft when the dressing was changed. The skin was taken between two fingers, and a phlebotomy scalpel was used to excise a thin skin fragment measuring 3–4 mm^2. Bleeding was usually limited to a single droplet.

Reverdin held that this method of obtaining skin grafts was not painful, and to illustrate this to his patients he occasionally excised a fragment of his own skin. The fragment taken in this demonstration was likewise used for the patient! Most surgeons preferred the medial aspect of the upper arm as donor site, because this is hairless (Dobson 1870 b, c; Lamm 1870; Steele 1870; Page 1870; Wood 1871; Gillespie 1871; Heiberg 1871 b, Boeck 1872). For the same reason, others obtained skin from the thigh (Morales 1871; Kappeler 1871). Other sites also served as donor sites, e.g. the forearm, the chest (Bryant 1872), the abdomen (Mason 1870 a) and the back of the hand (Netolitzky 1871).

The general opinion was that any part of the body could be considered as a donor site (Pollock 1871; Weiss 1872). In the selection of the donor site, the patient's wishes were respected. The patient usually preferred a site where the scar would be least conspicuous. In a period when skin grafting did not attract much attention, after 1874; Fischer (1880) proposed performing skin grafting in a bloodless fied and stretching the donor area to facilitate cutting the graft.

Simple instruments were used to obtain skin grafts. Forceps were usually used to lift the skin, and scissors were used to cut the skin beneath the forceps (Pollock 1870 d; Steele 1870; Page 1870; Czerny 1870; Gillespie 1871; Ranke, 1871; Kappeler 1871; Weiss 1872; Menzel 1872). Sometimes the central part of a graft thus obtained subsequently became necrotic. This is why several surgeons advised the use of delicate surgical forceps to lift the skin, to avoid bruising (Heiberg and Schulz 1871; Jacenko 1871 b; Hamilton 1871; Nehse 1872; Weiss 1872).

The case history presented by Boeck in 1872 illustrates that it was not always forceps that were applied too forcefully. He used to grasp the skin between his fingers when cutting the graft. On one occasion he had to pinch so forcefully (because the patient tried to pull his arm away) that he obtained a graft which, after application, developed necrosis in its centre.

Occasionally, a scalpel was used to remove a skin fragment (Mesterton 1871; Goldie 1871 a; Lesser 1873): the graft was then separated from the underlying structures with a single sweep. Hodgen (1871) and later Levis (1874) described a more elegant and less traumatic method of obtaining skin grafts. A thin needle with a handle was passed through a fold of skin. The needle was then lifted, with the skin, and the skin was cut along the needle with a rapid sawing motion, avoiding further damage to the skin (see Fig. 4). Ollier (1872 a, b), who used relatively large

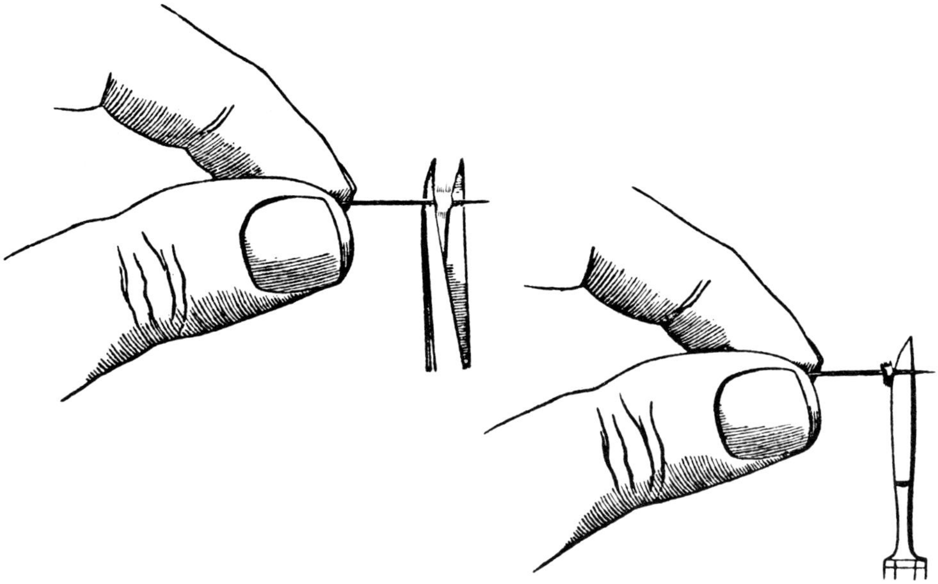

Fig. 4. The technique of cutting skin grafts could be facilitated with simple instruments such as needles by which the skin was lifted (Levis 1874)

skin grafts (4–8 cm²), obtained them with the aid of a cataract scalpel according to Beer or Richter (Poncet 1871). As early as 1871 it was found that a razor (still being used today) was a suitable instrument for this purpose (Netolitzky 1871; Mesterton 1871). Razors were also used at an early stage in Thiersch's department in Leipzig (Thierfelder 1872; Thiersch 1874). In view of the great interest taken in skin grafting during the early 1870s, it is not surprising that efforts were made to evolve instruments which might facilitate excision of skin grafts. In the *Lancet* of June 1871, such an instrument was described, not without pride, by its inventor Ferguson (1871 a, b). The instrument was called "forceps-scissors" (see Fig. 5).

It could be used single-handed to grasp and excise a skin fragment in one movement. The very next issue of the *Lancet* contained a letter to the editor by Macleod (1871 a), professor of surgery at the university of Glasgow, stating that he

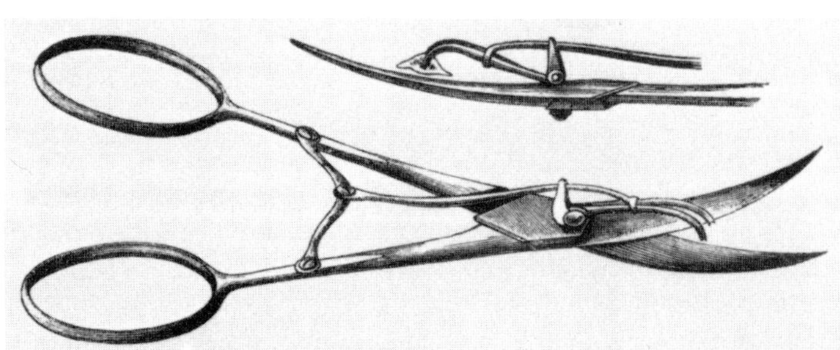

Fig. 5. The forceps-scissors were in use as a simple instrument to cut skin grafts. This instrument was presented in an article by Beigel (1872)

had recommended exactly the same instrument for the same purpose as early as April 1871 in the *British Medical Journal.*

He added that this instrument had been used in France for years to open fistulae. The forceps-scissors never became very popular; few surgeons used them (Bryant 1872; Weiss 1872; Beigel 1872).

When the great interest taken in skin grafting waned rapidly, because of the disappointing results, a few years after Reverdin's discovery, no further suggestions for new instruments appeared. The only exception was a scalpel with a blunt tip designed by August Reverdin (1876), a cousin of Jaques-Louis (see Fig. 6).

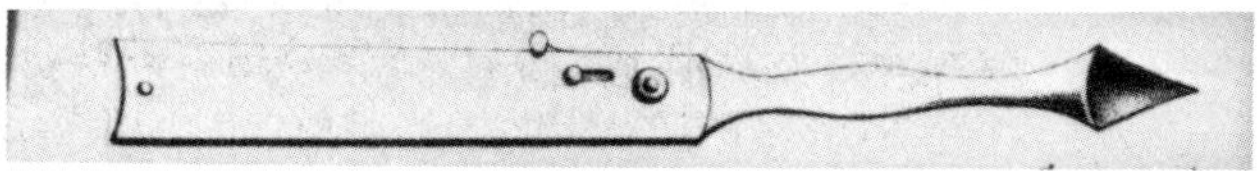

Fig. 6. The scalpel with a blunt tip to facilitate excision of pieces of skin advised by A. Reverdin (1876)

Most surgeons considered excision of a skin graft to be painless; possibly they did not notice the pain reaction of their patients. Nevertheless, patients regularly refused grafting because they were afraid of the pain. In a number of such cases, painlessness was then ensured by local or general anaesthesia. Kappeler (1871) of the *Kantonspital* in Münsterlingen, Switzerland, was among the authors who advocated local anaesthesia, but unfortunately he did not mention which anaesthetic he used. Wood (1871) used an ether spray – probably the ether apparatus of Richardson (Wiercx van Rhijn 1874).

Initially he was concerned about possible permanent damage to the tissues as a result of freezing, but this proved not to occur. Wood mentioned the following advantages of using an ether spray: the patient felt no pain and, because the skin was frozen, the surgeons could cut the grafts as thick as they wished. Ollier (1872 a + b) froze the donor site with a mixture of salt and ice to prevent pain. Procaine and cocaine were not yet available for local infiltration anaesthesia. General anaesthesia was also used. Ranke (1871), at that time chief of the children's out-patient clinic in Munich, described its application in a patient with burns which required skin grafting under general anaesthesia. Watson (1871) described his experience with repeated chloroform inhalation to anaesthetize a child with burns; during one of the many operations, the child developed respiratory arrest, and died. Henne (1874) likewise used chloroform. When he used homografts, a subject which will be discussed later, he anaesthetized the donor as well.

Nature of the Grafts

From the modern literature the impression is sometimes gained that, after Reverdin's first publication, grafts of one particular type and of particular dimensions and thickness were used and that, say, the full-thickness skin graft was not employed until much later.

This is far from true! From the very beginning, efforts were made to find that type of skin graft which ensured the best results. Investigations into optimal dimensions and thickness of grafts focused especially on the graft's ability to take.

Attempts were made with skin from other individuals, human as well as animal. In addition other surgeons tried to discover new sources of epithelium with which the objective – rapid healing of skin defects – could also be achieved. The quality of the cicatrix was a secondary consideration in these studies. In the next section the dimensions of the autografts and their thickness will be discussed. The use of epithelial grafts, homografts and heterografts will be discussed in separate sections.

Dimensions and Thickness of the Grafts

The first graft which Reverdin performed (1869) was done with skin fragments of about 1 mm^2. Later, he started using pieces of 3–4 mm^2 (Reverdin 1872). He cut these grafts as thin as possible because he was convinced that the epidermis made the principal contribution to wound healing. The defects which Reverdin was dealing with were on the whole ulcers. To him wound healing was synonymous with epithelialization. He considered the corium to be of subordinate importance. His sole criterion was that the graft should contain the Malpighian layer. Since it was virtually impossible to excise only epidermis without including part of the corium, which contained the capillaries, some slight bleeding usually occurred at the donor site. Reverdin described his grafts as "epidermic grafts" in order to indicate that the epidermis was the essential part of the graft; not, as many have since suggested, because he thought that the graft consisted solely of epidermis. At his very first presentation Reverdin was censured for having misjudged the thickness of his grafts (Desprès 1869) – a reproach which was repeated many times. The proceedings of the meeting clearly show, however, that Reverdin refuted this assertion. He had several reasons for using small grafts. Cutting small grafts caused no pain and the tiny size of the wounds reduced the risk of infection. However, the principal argument to prefer small grafts to larger ones was that many small grafts together had a much larger circumference from which epithelialization may occur than a single graft of the same size as the small grafts put together. Reverdin explicitly embraced the principle of surface enlargement.

Efforts to transplant larger pieces of skin were frequently attempted but generally failed. The principle of grafting was the same in all these cases, i.e. to apply epithelial islands. The dimensions of the grafts were generally defined exactly in the publications of this time. The size ranged from microscopical fragments (Lindenbaum 1871; Jacenko 1871 a, b) to fragments with a diameter of 3 cm (Heiberg 1871 a). The surface area of the latter does not differ very much from that of the grafts used by Ollier (1872 a + b).

Ollier used grafts with a surface area of 4–8 cm^2. His aim was quite different from that of Reverdin. His was not to create epithelial islands, but to cover defects completely with skin. On the basis of the dimensions of the skin fragments excised, they can be roughly divided into four categories:

a) Skin fragments with a diameter of less than 0.5 cm; the authors usually compared the dimensions with various agricultural products: Mason (1870 b) described the fragments as having the size of canary seed, Bryant (1872) as half the size of hemp seed, Howard (1871) as rice, Brown (1879) as oats, and Heath (1870), Arnott (1870), Tait (1870) and Goldie (1871 a) as split peas (see Fig. 7).

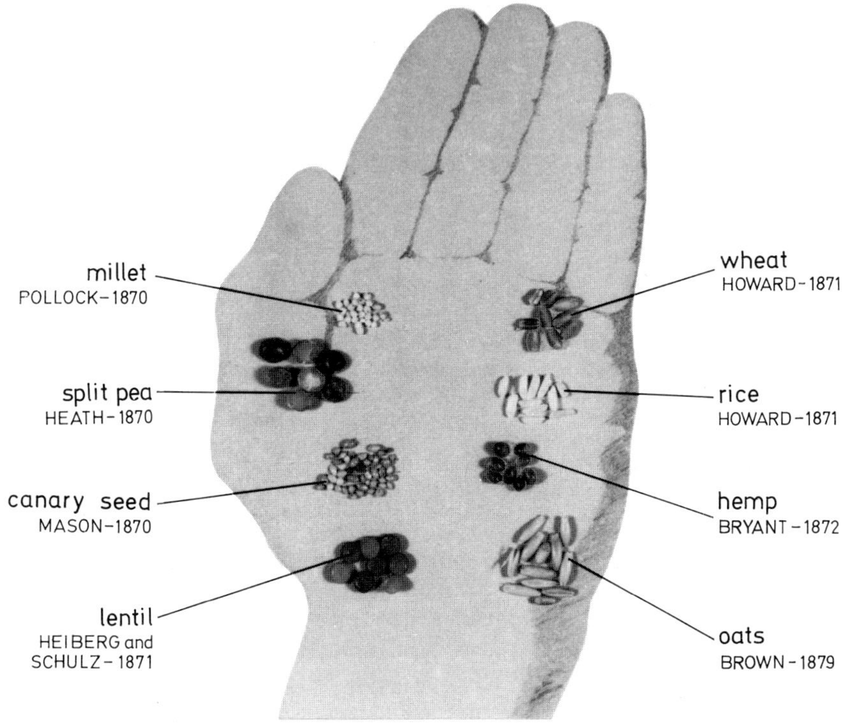

Fig. 7. The sizes of skin grafts were often compared with various kinds of seeds

b) Skin fragments with a diameter of about 0.5 cm were recommended by such authors as Johnson Smith (1870), Croft (1870), Page (1870), Gillespie (1871), Guipon (1874) and Coombs (1876).
c) Skin fragments with a diameter of 1–2 cm were used by Jacenko (1871 a, b), Macleod (1871 b), Busch (1872), Lindh (1872), Weiss (1872), Donnelly (1872), Menzel (1872), Anger (1874), Paci (1875) and Schede (1881).
d) Large grafts as were used by Ollier and Heiberg. Without doubt Fischer (1880) made use of the largest grafts which were as large as the object carrier of a microscope (diameter 10 cm).

It should not be concluded that the bigger pieces of skin were applied as such. Most surgeons divided them into even smaller ones for grafting. They were placed on the thumbnail and cut into smaller pieces. Kappeler (1871) was as more careful and placed the fragments on a cork for cutting. One of the principal reasons for division was that smaller fragments attached themselves more easily to the granulating surface (Dobson 1870 a, b; Wood 1871; Rodriguez 1871; Donnelly 1872; Macleod 1873; Woodman 1873; Wiercx van Rhijn 1874; McCarthy 1881).

The surgeons who performed skin transplantation soon discovered that the thickness of the graft was of great importance. As a rule, the purpose of the operation determined the graft thickness. Some preferred "thin" grafts; even these surgeons were aware, however, that the Malpighian layer should always be included in the graft, because a cicatricial island could form only in its presence (Page 1870; Dobson 1870 a, b; Steele 1870; Macleod 1871; Pollock 1871; Anderson 1871, Bryant 1872).

It was soon understood that a correlation existed between the rate of epithelialization and the graft thickness. Ash (1870) was among those who investigated this relation. He concluded that the thinner the grafts (i.e. the less corium was present), the more quickly a zone of epithelium formed round the graft. He also noticed that split-skin grafts sometimes attached themselves to wound surfaces which had failed to hold full-thickness grafts.

A study by Anderson (1871) revealed that grafts consisting solely of epidermis (he probably meant only the upper layers of the epidermis without the basal layer) or of full-thickness skin, either did not become the centre of an epithelial island, or did so much less rapidly than grafts which were thin but did contain the basal layer.

Some surgeons, however, opted in favour of full-thickness skin grafts (Lawson 1870 a, b, c, d; Woodman 1871; Howard 1871; Donnelly 1872; Weiss 1872; Boeck 1872; Henne 1874). Donnelly argued that growth of epithelium was possible only if the graft contained corium, because the epidermis detached itself spontaneously after skin grafting. This was why, in his opinion, the epidermis could not play a role in epithelialization. Donnelly probably assumed that the entire epidermis detached itself.

Heiberg (1871 a, b) probably also used full-thickness skin, although he did not specifically mention this. He reported favourable results, but alas, only short-term ones. The donor sites were closed with sutures because otherwise it might take months before the sites healed.

Every surgeon who used full-thickness skin grafts was convinced that the subcutaneous fat had to be carefully removed because otherwise the grafts would not, or only insufficiently, become attached to the wound surface (Woodman 1871; Jacenko 1871 b; Lindenbaum 1871; Bryant 1872; Weiss 1872; Menzel 1872) (Fig. 8). Peet (1977) mistakenly assumes that Wolfe (1875) was the first to under-

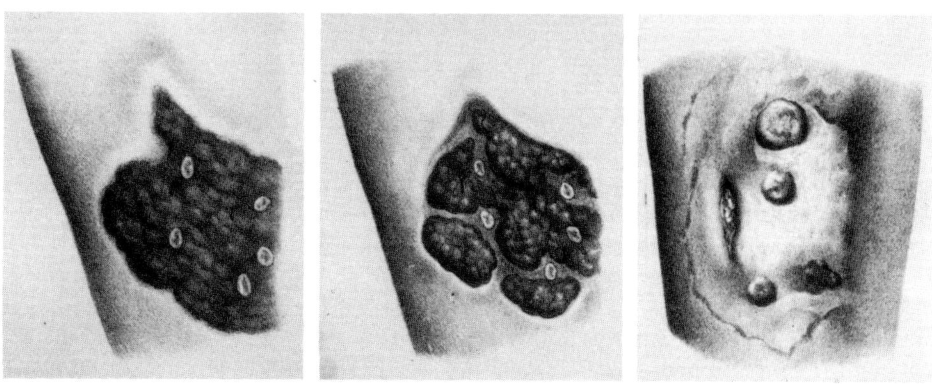

Fig. 8. Healing of a wound by skin grafts, shown in three phases. Illustrations from an article of Bryant (1872)

stand the importance of removing the subcutaneous fat. Today, this important rule in full-thickness skin grafting is still observed. The celebrated French surgeon Ollier (1872 a + b), as already described, made a sawing movement when cutting relatively large grafts, with a surface area of 4–8 cm^2. At the periphery, these grafts were thin and consisted only of epidermis; the centre consisted of full-thickness skin, sometimes even with a layer of subcutaneous fat (if so, the fat was removed). Ollier prefered to use full-thickness grafts because they yielded the best qualitative results. He covered tissue defects with grafts as best he could, in order to prevent secondary epithelialization, as has been discussed previously. He maintained that there was no difference in quality between scars after healing by second intention and those after application of skin grafts consisting mainly of epidermis.

For large granulating surfaces, several small grafts were as a rule used in order to obtain the largest possible number of islands of epithelialization (Pollock 1871; Anderson 1871; Reverdin 1872). In functionally less important areas, fewer grafts were applied than in areas of greater functional importance. It was advised that ulcers of the leg be treated with numerous full-thickness grafts of fair size in order to ensure an optimal quality (particularly elasticity) and to avoid contraction as far as possible (Steele 1870; Heiberg 1871 b). For the operative correction of contractures, Anderson (1871) of St. Thomas' Hospital in London, also used grafts of the largest possible size. Thiersch (1874) used full-thickness grafts in his studies of wound healing after skin grafting. This discussion about the optimal size and thickness of the grafts was after all not so important, because after 1874 the interest in skin grafting among general surgeons disappeared.

Application of the Grafts

The grafts were simply placed on red, firm granulating surfaces (Rodriguez 1871) or carefully pressed on (Dobson 1870 b; Bryant 1872). This was usually done with bare hands, but a needle was occasionally also used. The needle was then used to move the graft to-and-fro until the edges, which tended to curl, were in direct contact with the underlying structures (Dobson 1870 b; Weiss 1872). In some cases a small incision was made in the granulation tissue, whereupon the graft was placed in the defect (Editorial 1870 a; Johnson Smith 1870; Anderson 1871; Kappeler 1871). Reverdin is often mentioned as the first surgeon to use this variant, but he himself wrote that he had done this in only one case (Reverdin 1872). In his opinion, this method was indicated only if the granulation tissue was of poor quality. Czerny (1870), who a year later at the age of 29 was appointed professor of surgery in Freiburg, investigated the possible advantages of inserting grafts in granulation tissue. He found that when the grafts were placed *on* the granulation tissue, the epithelial zone nine days later was larger than after *in*sertion of the grafts. After two weeks, the zones were the same size in either case. Pollock (1871) and Hamilton (1871) reached the same conclusion. Hamilton (1871) went even further and observed that "... it does not seem to be a matter of any consequence how the graft is laid, whether with the raw turned in one direction or the other." In this context it should be noted that Hamilton used very small grafts. Howard (1871) not only incised the granulation tissue but in fact removed a fragment, thus creating a depression in which the graft fitted snugly. The grafts were generally fixed in position with a dressing. Only North (1886) reported that he made use of a suture which he passed through the graft and the granulation tissue. It is difficult to understand how he succeeded in getting enough support in this tissue.

In application of the grafts, the question arose of how far they should be placed from the wound edges. As already mentioned, it was known that the quality of the cicatrix was much better if the grafts were spaced closer together. In the first operation on skin defects in non-functional areas, the grafts were about 1 inch (2.5 cm) from each other (Steele 1870; Pollock 1871; Hamilton 1871; Bryant 1872).

The scar obtained in this way was of moderate quality, and the grafts were consequently spaced closer and closer together, until they were about 1 cm apart (McCarthy, 1881). When dressings were changed, the opportunity was often utilized to apply new grafts.

Steele (1870), surgeon at the Bristol Royal Infirmary, assumed that this had a favourable effect on the wound floor, because each new graft would stimulate the wound surface, bringing "... freshness and vigour to the whole surface". On the other hand, Nehse (1872) in his thesis (Berlin) cautioned against applying too many grafts. He compared this with the gardener who plants too many flower seeds, and thus impedes the full development of all the flowers! Fischer was a teacher in surgery in Strasbourg; his special place is not only illustrated by the fact that he advised the use of a bloodless operation field or that the skin should be stretched to simplify the cutting of grafts but also by his advising the use of incisions in the grafts to encourage drainage (Fischer 1880).

Dressing After Grafting

Wound care without dressing has hardly been described. Only A. Reverdin (1876) intimated that he sometimes left facial wounds uncovered. The grafted wounds were dressed, sometimes with simple dressings, but in other cases with complex multiple-layer dressings. Reverdin (1869) used a dressing with diachylon ointment (unguentum diachylon, made up of fifty parts lead plaster and fifty parts sesame oil). He did not mention why it was precisely diachylon that he used. Watson (1871), Dubrueil (1872), Menzel (1872) and Anger (1874) followed Reverdin's example. Poncet (1871) likewise used dressings with diachylon, but at the sites of the grafts he applied goldbeater's skin to prevent adhesion of the grafts to the dressing. The most popular dressing was that with adhesive plaster, which was often the sole material used to cover the wound. Adhesive plaster [4] was preferred by many, because it held the grafts well fixed in position (Editorial 1870 a; Fiddes 1870; Czerny 1870, 1871 a, b; Ranke 1871; Wood 1871; Macleod 1871 b; Anderson 1871; Morales 1871; Donnelly 1872; Busch 1872). However, adhesive plaster was used for other reasons also. The Russian surgeon, Jacenko (1871 a) believed that it softened the granulation tissue, which he regarded as an advantage.

Kappeler (1871) studied the properties of adhesive plaster in relation to other types of dressing, e.g. those with carbolic acid, chlorated water and camphor spirit. He concluded that the epithelial islands increased in size most rapidly beneath adhesive plaster. He did not suggest that the other agents might in fact inhibit

4 Emplastrum adhaesivum, made up of ten parts caoutchouc, twenty parts wool fat, and seventy parts lead plaster.

epithelialization. One of the disadvantages of adhesive plaster was that the course of wound healing could be assessed only after removal of the plaster. This rapidly led to the use of transparent dressings, which did not have to be changed so frequently. Examples were: transparent isinglass (Mason 1870 a; Page 1870; Lawson 1870 a, b, 1871; Jacenko 1871 a, b), Lister's varnish plaster (Dobson, 1870 c) and gutta-percha [5] (Steele 1870; Bryant 1872; Bligh 1873; Brown 1879). One of the major disadvantages of the various dressing materials was that the grafts stuck to them.

To prevent this, all sorts of agents were investigated, e.g. the goldbeater's skin that Poncet (1871) used. This was often used in surgery of the eyelids. Other examples of non-adhesive dressings were tinfoil paper (Menzel 1872), rubber paper (Nehse 1872) and gauze impregnated with carbolated oil, glycerin or some indifferent ointment (Rodriguez 1871; Forster 1872; Weiss 1872).

More complex multiple dressings gradually came to be used more and more, for two reasons: to keep the grafts warm, and to ensure better immobilization (Watson 1871; Lawson 1871; Wood 1871; Jacenko 1871 b; Lindenbaum 1871).

The method used by Steele (1870) is an instructive example. Gutta-percha was placed on the grafted wound; this was covered with a layer of dressing soaked in water or some other indifferent fluid, which in turn was covered with a cotton wool compress. A bandage was finally applied to ensure fixation. The cotton wool served to ensure immobilization and to keep the wound warm. Lindenbaum stressed that a circular bandage had to be applied if at all possible, because this ensured optimal immobilization. The wet dressings were sometimes also used to reduce suppuration (Anderson 1871). Heiberg and Schulz were probably the first to suggest the use of padding to ensure adequate immobilization (Heiberg 1871 b; Heiberg and Schulz 1871). This suggestion was immediately accepted by Weiss (1872) and Lochner (1872). The technique was as follows: the grafts were covered with adhesive plaster or transparent English plaster, on which a wad of cotton wool was then placed, which in turn was fixed with adhesive plaster. It was generally agreed that immobilization was an important prerequisite for a successful outcome. In addition to dressings, other aids such as splints were used to ensure immobilization (Coulson 1871; Hofmokl 1871). Hofmokl used wooden splints. Ollier (1872 b) used a special splint, of which unfortunately he gave no description. Sometimes wire cages were used to protect grafted areas (Fischer 1880). Few data could be found on the length of time during which a limb was immobilized after grafting. Woodman (1871) prescribed a few days' bed rest for patients treated by grafting of an ulcer of the leg. Other surgeons also prescribed bed rest, but failed to specify how long (Macleod 1871 b; Hamilton 1871; Wurfbain 1871; Lochner 1872). In practice it became apparent that it was very difficult to submit the patients with grafted ulcers of the leg to a regime of rest. When the patients saw that the wounds were closed they did not accept further immobilization and left their beds. The only author to discuss postoperative management in some detail was Parish (1872) of Philadelphia. He prescribed bed rest and later, when his patients were allowed to sit in a chair, the leg had to be kept horizontal. Until healing was complete, his patients were not

5 Gummi plasticum depuratum, made up of the coagulated milky juice obtained from the leaves and the trunk of various species of the genus *Palaquium* and some related Sapotacieae.

allowed to walk or stand. By "healing", Parish probably meant the process of epithelialization by which the wound closed. He was the only one to define his understanding of wound healing. It may well be that the too brief period of rest prescribed after grafting was one of the reasons why results were so often disappointing. To prevent injuries and swelling of the leg, after transplantation Fischer (1880) prescribed elastic bandages for his patients.

The First Wound Inspection

Premature and too-frequent inspection of grafted wounds was considered to be harmful. Nevertheless, several surgeons inspected the wounds on the very first day after operation (Reverdin 1869; Storch 1871; Weiss 1872; Nehse 1872). Later, Reverdin (1872) changed his policy and waited four days before inspecting the wounds. No consensus was achieved about the best time for the first wound inspection. The literature indicates, however, that the tendency was to inspect between the second and the fourth postoperative days. [6]

Consequences of Grafting

The Reaction of the Wound

The surgeons were impressed by the phenomenon of epithelium formation around grafts, but were especially surprised that the epithelium grew mostly in the direction of other grafts, or towards the nearest wound edge. As soon as the grafts attached themselves, the wound edges began to epithelialize (Steele 1870). Anderson (1871) in fact regarded epithelialization from the wound edges as the first sign of acceptance of the grafts. The wound edge showed increased growth of epithelium in the direction of the grafts (Reverdin 1869). The grafts apparently promoted epithelialization from the wound edges (Coulson 1871; Barlow 1870; Pollock 1871; Storch 1871; Heiberg and Schultz 1871; Bryant 1871; Kappeler 1871; Ranke 1871; Reverdin 1871 a, b; Pooley 1871).

The closer to the wound edges the grafts were placed, the more the epithelialization was stimulated (Bryant 1872; Weiss 1872). Dobson (1870 a) tried to objectify this phenomenon in a more or less comparative study. In a patient with two virtually identical ulcers of the leg, grafts were placed on the granulation tissue of one ulcer, while the other ulcer received no grafts. The ulcers were otherwise treated in exactly the same way. The edges of the grafted ulcer changed; they lost their whitish, sharply indurated appearance. The edges of the non-grafted ulcer did not change. Dobson was unable to explain this. Bogg (1870) believed that grafts attracted specific "skin blood", which promoted healing at the site of the grafts and the wound edges. He did not specify what he meant by "skin blood".

---

6 The lack of consensus is illustrated by the following data. Inspection of the wound was carried out after two days by Dobson (1870 b), Steele (1870), Page (1870), Kappeler (1871) and Hamilton (1871); after three days by Johnson Smith (1870), Lawson (1870 b), Heiberg and Schulz (1871) and Bryant (1872); and after four days by Fiddes (1870), Rodriguez (1871), Jacenko (1871 b), Busch (1872), Lochner (1872) and Lindh (1872). Pollock (1871) set no fixed time for the first wound inspection; in some cases he left the dressings in situ as long as ten days.

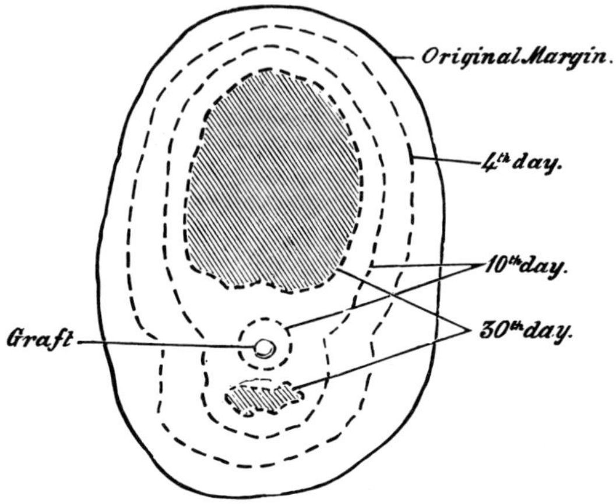

Fig. 9. One of the first illustrations in which the stimulation of epithelialization from the edges of the wound by a skin graft is shown. The hatched area is not yet covered with epithelium thirty days after grafting (Anderson 1871)

The Reaction of the Grafts

The behaviour of the grafts in the wound was carefully studied. Reverdin (1869) observed that "epidermis" formed around the graft six days after grafting. The zones of "epidermis" around individual grafts merged as soon as they touched.

The grafts did not always show the same behaviour. In fact it was sometimes difficult to trace a graft a few days after its application (Johnson Smith 1870; Hamilton 1871). When the graft did remain identifiable it was first white and pale (Lawson 1871; Lindenbaum 1871). After two days it assumed a pinkish colour (Jacenko 1871 a, b). At that time the graft adhered to the underlying structures (Lindenbaum 1871). After two to four days the superficial layer of the graft detached itself (Anderson 1871; Kappeler 1871; Lesser 1873). Why it did so remained obscure. Pollock (1870 c) thought that the layer detached itself because it had fulfilled its task. In that part of the graft that remained intact, circulation was restored. Steele (1870) and Lindenbaum (1871) observed that a narrow bluish zone appeared around the graft before the fifth day. Most surgeons did not see this thin, greyish layer of epithelium until after five to eight days. Once it appeared, it rapidly spread (Dobson 1870 c; Anderson 1871; Kappeler 1871; Reverdin 1872; Weiss 1872).

Not all grafts showed an active tendency to form epithelium. In some, no epithelial zone formed; in others, the formation of this zone took a very long time; in yet others, the zone remained limited to a very narrow strip. The differences in graft behaviour were, Lindenbaum (1871) thought, due to differences in the quality of the wound floor and the grafts themselves. Thin grafts adhered more readily than thick ones, and formed epithelial zones more quickly.

Wound Healing After Skin Grafting

Two facets of wound healing after skin grafting received particular attention: The question of how the graft could survive on the wound bed and why an epithelial zone formed around the graft. The investigations into these two questions were based on clinical observations and microscopic findings. One of the first to formulate theories on wound healing after skin grafting was the Russian surgeon Lindenbaum (1871). His theory was based on the postulate that grafting could only be done successfully on a granulating wound surface; consequently, "The presence of granulation tissue had to be a factor in healing." He assumed that fresh wounds were covered with a layer of necrotic tissue, while granulation tissue was not. In granulation tissue, he reasoned, the blood vessels extended into the top layer of the most superficial part. The distance between the vessels in the granulation tissue and the graft was only small. Lindenbaum (1871) therefore assumed that the survival of grafts was based on restoration of the circulation.

A few years later, Thiersch (1874) addressed a meeting of the *Deutsche Gesellschaft für Chirurgie* to report the results of his extensive studies on graft healing. At the time Thiersch was already well known for his expertise in the use of contrast media to visualize the microcirculation. (More biografical information about Thiersch follows in Chap. 4.) He had studied a patient whose leg was to be amputated. The patient had an ulcer of the leg, which continued to relapse in spite of several Reverdin skin grafts. The patient finally requested an amputation. On several occasions prior to the amputation, full-thickness skin grafts with a surface area of 1 cm^2 were excised from the vicinity of the ulcer, and applied to its granulating surface. The last graft was applied 18 hours before amputation. Wound healing was studied in several stages, visualizing the microcirculation by the injection technique which Thiersch had evolved. He was able to demonstrate a vascular communication between the wound bed and the graft applied 18 hours previously. The vessels of the wound bed communicated with intercellular spaces in the graft, which according to Thiersch acted as some kind of primitive blood vessels. These spaces were converted to real blood vessels within a few days. Thiersch was unable to identify the sites at which the capillaries of the wound bed entered the graft. In the grafts applied two weeks before amputation, complete integration between the vascular systems of wound bed and graft had occurred. The capillaries gradually became wider, extended and assumed a meandering, curly course. Thiersch described these features as "embryonic". The capillaries had resumed a normal appearance three to four weeks after grafting. Thiersch assumed that an entirely new capillary system developed in the graft. He was unable to identify the fibrin layer between graft and granulation tissue, which other surgeons (Weiss 1872) had mentioned. Only exceptionally did the entire thickness of the graft remain intact.

The frequently observed shedding of the superficial layer of the graft was due, Thiersch thought, to insufficient circulation during the period after grafting. He concluded that the corium constituted an important part of the graft. After full-thickness skin grafting, a layer which comprised the entire epidermis and papillary layer sometimes detached itself. In those cases the epithelial remnants of the intact sudoriferous glands ensured epithelialization.

In 1872 Thierfelder, who worked in Thiersch's department, had already published some findings on wound healing after grafting.

He had studied wound healing three weeks after homografting in one patient, and two months after autografting in another. Unfortunately he did not specify the dimensions and thickness of the grafts used. Examining a biopsy specimen from the cicatrix of a homograft performed three weeks earlier, Thierfelder observed a fibrin layer between wound bed and graft. This layer comprised many cells and blood vessels, but only a few connective tissue fibres. In the (homo)graft, old as well as new blood vessels were found. The old vessels were as a rule thrombotic. The epidermis with the Malpighian layer presented a normal appearance. Thierfelder concluded that the grafted skin was connected to the underlying structures via blood vessels. In the biopsy specimen from the patient examined two months after autografting, a thin horny layer and a normal Malpighian layer with flat papillae were found; a fibrin layer was no longer identifiable between graft and wound bed. This bed comprised spaces which were also present in the graft, and which often contained round cells. Thiersch and Thierfelder while coming from the same department came to different conclusions.

While some surgeons were convinced of the importance of circulation between graft and wound bed, others attached but little importance to it (Dobson 1870 b; Reverdin 1871 a, b, 1872). Reverdin believed that grafts attach themselves to the underlying structures in two phases. In the first, by activities of epithelial cells, because he had observed at microscopic examination that epithelial cells from the graft edges moved as club-like protrusions along the undersurface of the grafts and the wound floor, thus enclosing the corium part of the grafts by epithelial cells. The formation of epithelial cells took place from the deep layers of the epidermis. Only in the second phase did Reverdin observe communication via blood vessels between wound floor and graft. He, too, described the blood vessels observed in the grafts in the initial phase, as "embryonic" vessels. Apart from the microscopic findings Reverdin had other reasons to consider the circulation to be of subordinate importance. He had noticed that grafts which failed to attach themselves to the underlying tissue did sometimes adhere to the underlying tissue at some other sites. Their vitality, therefore, remained intact. Reverdin assumed that grafts could survive by virtue of the fluid formed by granulation tissue. Lesser (1873) likewise mentioned the importance of this fluid.

At microscopic examination, Reverdin found that grafted skin began to resemble "embryonic" tissue more and more closely. In the corium, most of the elastic fibres disappeared. He regarded this as an important finding because the quality of the grafted tissue largely depended on the amount of elastic fibres which remained intact. This is a remarkable statement by Reverdin, who again and again intimated that he regarded the epidermis as the essential structure of the graft, while in his opinion the corium was hardly important.

As already mentioned, studies on wound healing focussed on two aspects: (1) how the grafts could survive, and (2) how epithelialization around the graft developed. The almost unanimous opinion was that epithelialization in a graft always arose from the Malpighian layer. The cells formed by this layer fanned out over the granulation tissue. Pollock (1870 c) studied epithelialization with the aid of a magnifying glass. He saw that a thin transparent layer of tissue first formed around the graft. Initially he thought that this membrane contained a network of tiny blood vessels, but later he discovered that the blood vessels were localized beneath this thin epithelial layer. This thin zone lost its transparency within a few days, and assumed a white colour. The blood vessels seemed to disappear. The zone gradually increased in width, but also in thickness due to formation of epithelial cells from the depth towards the surface. In his opinion epithelial cells were made in the Malpighian layer. The cicatrix which resulted from the epithelialization of the small grafts did not contain more elastic fibres than obtained by healing from the wound edges, as he had hoped.

To his surprise Pollock observed that the shrinking which always accompanied secondary wound healing was not seen after grafting. The shortness of his period of observation may have played a role in this respect. Pollock was unable to establish whether the scar obtained after grafting contained sudoriferous glands. Golding Bird (1874) studied the changes which occurred in the granulation tissue while this was being covered with epithelium. Beneath the epithelium, the intercellular structure changed: connective tissue fibres formed, and the cells in the granulation tissue disappeared in large numbers. The speed of these changes depended on the growth of the epithelium. Anderson (1871) had previously described the conversion of granulation tissue to fibrous connective tissue beneath the epithelium. In spite of intensive efforts, Golding Bird failed to demonstrate this conversion. Coupland (1874) believed that the granulation tissue turned into epithelial tissue. In those days an important point of scientific discussion was whether new epithelium developed from epithelial cells in the transplants or from the wound bed. Although many disagreed completely with Coupland, his view was corroborated by Dobson (1870b), Johnson Smith (1870) and Reverdin (1871a, b, 1872).

We have already mentioned that Thierfelder (1872) used homografts in his studies on wound healing. This is not surprising in view of the fact that it was at that time almost generally accepted that autografts and homografts hardly differed. Several other investigators also used homografts in their studies. Pollock (Editorial 1870 a), for example, used homografts because he wondered whether pigmented epithelial cells could multiply in the same way as unpigmented cells. He therefore wanted to know what would happen when skin from a negro was grafted onto a granulating skin defect in a caucasian. This experiment was performed in June 1870. Two weeks after application of the dark skin graft, it increased in size; and after nine weeks a fair-sized dark area had developed, which was not evenly dark throughout. Pollock (1870 f) concluded that the cells in black skin equalled those in white skin as to reproducibility. In subsequent publications, however, Pollock (1870 b, c, e, f) reported that the dark pigmented tissue had been destroyed completely by some unknown process!

This study attracted considerable attention in the British medical world, because it raised the question whether experiments in which black skin was grafted onto white persons were ethically acceptable (Pollock 1870 a, d, e).

Dark pigmented skin was used also in an effort to find the answer to the important and principal question whether proliferation of epithelial cells arose from the grafted skin or from the wound surface.

Bryant (1872), a surgeon at Guy's Hospital, grafted black skin onto granulation tissue of an ulcer of the leg in a white patient. In the course of ten weeks, the homografts grew to twenty times their original size. Together they formed a single, large, dark area (see Fig. 8), and in Bryant's opinion this demonstrated that the proliferation of epithelial cells arose from the grafts.

Johnson Smith (1870) and Reverdin (1871 a, b, 1872) performed similar experiments. They, too, observed the development of a dark epithelial zone around

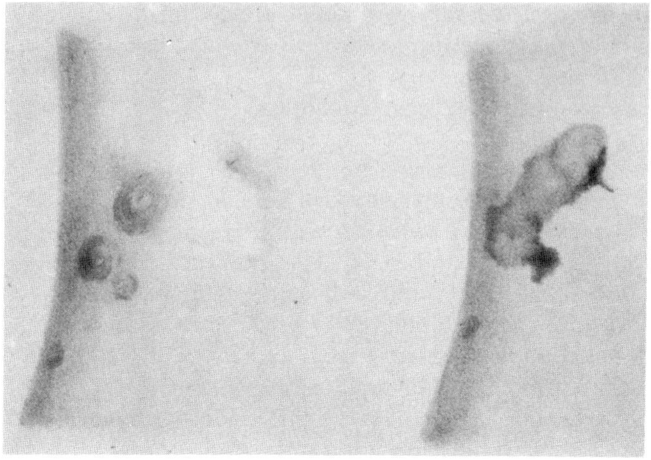

Fig. 10. The increase of the pigmented area of epithelium resulting from transplantation of black skin in a white patient (Bryant 1872)

the graft. The larger the zone became, the more the dark colour faded. They therefore concluded that cicatrization with the aid of grafts was not based on multiplication of the epithelial cells of the graft itself (for in that case the epithelial zone should have retained its dark colour as it increased in size), but on some other process. Maurel (1878) confirmed that black skin, when grafted onto a skin defect in a caucasian, lost its dark colour. He assumed that the "embryonic" tissue had only a limited ability to produce pigment.

On the other hand, white skin was used in grafts on negroes (Maxwell 1873). Maxwell (New Castle, Delaware) grafted a fragment of his own skin onto a granulating facial defect in a negro. The graft was accepted and increased in size. The area at first remained white, but gradually changed its colour and was entirely black (the cicatrix) after three months. Maxwell loosely explained this by assuming that skin colour is determined by the blood, and that the graft cells play no role in this respect.

Another question which attracted attention was whether skin from young individuals had better healing properties than that from aged people. In this context, Dobson (1870 b) grafted skin from a young man and skin from the patient himself onto a granulating wound in an old man. During a given period, the former graft formed a larger epithelial zone than the latter. Dobson did not mention how long he followed the wound healing. He did conclude that skin from young donors stimulated the growth of epithelium around grafts more intensively than skin from aged donors.

Dobson proceeded from the assumption that epithelial growth was started from the wound bed, the graft playing no role in this respect.

Results of Skin Grafting

Skin grafting became highly popular after its introduction by Reverdin (1869), and medical journals paid ample attention to this subject. Gradually, however, the interest waned, and in the years between 1874 and 1886 there were hardly any publications on free skin grafting. The principal reason for this change was that the results were disappointing. Several factors must have played a part here, e.g. wrong indications (ulcer of the leg), the grafting technique, the use of homografts and the postoperative management. The initial enthusiasm was based in part on very early reports of favourable results (Arnott 1870; Johnson Smith 1870). Surgeons who studied long-term results concluded that the tegument obtained after grafting did not differ from that obtained after healing by second intention. The scar was of moderate quality, and disrupted at the slightest provocation (Page 1870; Wilson 1870; Hamilton 1871; Lochner 1872; Studensky 1873; Hickl 1875). It was initially expected that skin grafts could prevent shrinking (Steele 1870; Macleod 1871 b; Nicholls 1871). Later, after years of careful observation, Hickl (1875) concluded that the same degree of shrinking occurred after skin grafting as after healing by second intention.

The cosmetic results were hardly mentioned in the first few years. They were not the principal objective of the operation. The primary purpose was to close skin defects. Menzel (1872) described the results as cosmetically poor. Years later, he was still able to identify the grafts as elevated islands. Moreover, they had a conspicuous, contrasting white colour. Ellipsoid grafts with a diameter of 1 cm caused the ugliest scars, and he therefore proposed that in cases where the appearance was important (e.g. in the face), very small grafts should be used, or on the contrary relatively large grafts, with a diameter of 2.5 cm.

Surgeons generally expressed optimism about sensory recovery, but no statements were made about the type of sensibility. Lawson (1870 b, c, d) recorded the quickest sensory recovery. He maintained that, within ten days of the operation, the patient could feel the graft when it was touched with a blunt object. It is to be noted that this was a graft on the upper eyelid. Jacenko (1871 b) held that tactile sensibility was restored within 15 days; Bryant (1872) confined himself to the remark that the sensibility of the scar was in any case better than in non-grafted areas. Others, like Kappeler (1871) and Weiss (1872) were more cautious; they could not determine exactly when sensibility returned, but they agreed that it took some considerable time, longer even than the period of five weeks which Heiberg and Schulz (1871) had suggested.

Although long-term results were scarcely reported, there is one description of a follow-up over several years. This concerned the patient on whom Pollock (1870 a, b, c, d, e, f) performed his first skin graft. She was a girl with old burns.

The wounds had healed five months after the first grafting (Pollock 1870 b). One year later this patient was again described by Haward (1871 a, b, c): at that time the grafted areas looked like normal skin, but without hairs. The more numerous the grafts that had been applied to a given area, the more closely the scar resembled normal skin. One year after the operation the girl was in a good condition. Movements could be normally executed with the burnt leg. In 1873 (three years after treatment) the *Lancet* published a special unsigned note on the same girl, who had been hospitalized for other reasons. The scars on the leg were in good condition. "The new tissue extending from the nates down the back of the thigh to below the knee shows low tendency to contract and possesses sensibility" (Pollock, 1873).

Apart from this favourable report it was not difficult to find reports of poor results. These were described especially in patients with ulcers of the leg. These usually relapsed as soon as the patient was allowed to go about again (Lawson 1871; Bryant 1872; Levis 1874; Thiersch 1874). The erroneous impression might be gained that surgeons at the time did not know that an ulcer of the leg can be a result of another disease. Kappeler (1871) had treated 15 patients with varicose ulcers. After grafting, the ulcers healed more quickly than after conservative treatment; however, he observed relapses because, he maintained, he could not properly treat the venous insufficiency. As far as could be discovered Kappeler was the only one who tried to explain the poor results in the treatment of ulcers. He did notice that relapses occurred sooner in conservatively treated patients than in those who had received grafts. As a rule when the ulcers relapsed, the grafts themselves remained intact. Lawson (1871) had made similar observations and therefore advised the use of several large full-thickness skin grafts in treating ulcers of the leg. In ulcers of the leg grafting results would continue to be disappointing, even when new methods of grafting were introduced decades later.

B. The Grafting of Epithelium Without Corium

After Reverdin's invention intensive studies were made of the thickness and dimensions of the grafts which would give the best results. These studies nearly always proceeded from the assumption that the graft should in any case contain the Malpighian layer. Some surgeons, however, studied the question whether epithelial cells not attached to other skin layers could be grafted.

Epithelial Scrapings

Small fragments of epithelium, obtained by scraping the skin, might perhaps be grafted. This possibility was investigated at an early date, and continued to be the subject of later studies. Fiddes (Editorial 1870 c) is generally considered to have been the first to use epithelial scrapings on skin defects. He probably was not. Fiddes reported his attempts on 17th December 1870 in the *Lancet*, in a letter to the editor, dated 5th December 1870 (Fiddes 1870). But on 25th June 1870 the French surgeon de Ranse (1870) had published in the *Gazette médicale de Paris* the proceedings of a meeting of the *Société de Chirurgie de Paris*, during which Marc Sée (1870) had read a paper on skin grafting in which epithelial scrapings were also mentioned: "... A few days later he (Marc Sée) performed another graft by placing on the wound surface some particles of epidermis obtained by scraping the surface of the arm with a lancet." An almost literal translation of de Ranse's report appeared in *The British Medical Times and Gazette* of 9th July 1870. Fiddes had formed the conviction that only some fragments of epithelial tissue were required to ensure cicatrization of a skin defect and on the basis of this conviction he believed that cicatrization could be stimulated enormously by applying numerous minute particles of epithelium to the wound surface. He chose epidermal scrapings as a source of epithelial particles. These scrapings were obtained by scraping the convex part of a limb with a knife held perpendicular to the skin. The data supplied by Fiddes did not indicate to what depth the skin was scraped; apparently his scrapings remained very superficial. Certainly not so deep as to cause bleeding. The scrapings which adhered to the knife, were strewn over a granulating surface and kept in position with adhesive plaster. Three to four days later the wound surface had assumed a glassy, bluish appearance. According to Fiddes, a scar finally formed which had the appearance and the quality of normal skin!

Fiddes assumed that the scrapings were dry epithelial cells which still contained a nucleus. He believed that the dried cells imbibed the serum secreted by the granulation tissue, thus undergoing some sort of revitalization.

Although Nicholls (1871) and Hodgen (1871) corroborated the favourable results with epithelial scrapings, other surgeons maintained that the dead cells of the superficial epidermal layer made no contribution whatsoever to cicatrization (Ash 1870; Jacenko 1871 b). They proposed that the deeper layers of epidermis should also be used for this purpose. Several surgeons studied the question whether epidermal scrapings could influence the speed of wound healing. The results were uniformly poor (Goldie 1871 b; Rodriguez 1871; Pooley 1871; Czerny 1871 b; Kappeler 1871; Bryant 1872; Lesser 1873; Levis 1874; Schweninger 1875; Leale 1878).

Macleod (1871 b) also obtained disappointing results with this method, but he noticed that the scrapings did seem to have an unexpectedly favourable effect on the wound edges. The epithelialization from the wound edges seemed to be stimulated. He made no mention of the possibility that factors other than the epithelial scrapings might influence epithelialization, e.g. a different way of dressing the wound. Other authors were in fact unable to corroborate his observation.

Warts

An original attempt to influence circatrization was made by the New-Yorker Leale (1878). He believed that warts might be an important source of epithelium because they consisted of a thick layer of epidermis. Epithelialization, he reasoned, might be vigorously stimulated by grafting fragments of warts. In a patient with burns who also had warts, he removed several of these warts, cut them into small fragments and applied these to the granulating surface. All fragments had attached themselves within 48 hours. Three weeks later the defect was closed and covered by a firm scar. Leale's idea elicited few reactions, although a few years later Pilcher (1881) remarked that he preferred warts (epithelium) to skin grafts.

Hair Roots

Schweninger (1875), assistant in the institute of pathology in Munich, proceeded from the assumption that hair roots contain epithelial cells with proliferative properties. He wondered whether this source of epithelium could be used to accelerate the healing of skin defects. Consequently he "grafted" hairs pulled out with their roots, onto granulating tissues. He observed that an epithelial (cicatricial) island with a diameter of 2 mm formed around the hair root within three to five days. These islands gradually increased in size, but remained within certain limits. Schweninger concluded that the epithelial cells in the outer layers of the hair roots could produce epithelial cells in granulating surfaces. He did not express himself about the practical value of "hair root grafting". His investigations received very little attention.

C. Homografting

Skin grafting flourished soon after Reverdin's invention, but subsequently lost its popularity almost as quickly. Its rapid rise was probably based on evaluation of short-term results. Long-term results proved to be much less favourable. In some cases they were in fact very disappointing. One of the principal reasons for these disappointing results must have been that autografts and homografts were used indiscriminately, as indicated by Reverdin (1872) who wrote:

"... in my first grafts I used skin from the patient himself, but I soon became convinced that the result was the same when I used skin from another individual. This has been demonstrated with certainty." This statement was corroborated by several authors (Steele 1870; Anderson 1871; Macleod 1871 b; Heiberg and Schulz 1871; Bardeleben 1874; Hill 1875; Lloyd 1876; Paci 1875; Fischer 1880).

The conviction that autografts and homografts produced the same results was so strong that publications in the 1870s scarcely mentioned the particular type of graft used. [7]

Another illustration of the alleged equality of the two types of graft lies in the fact that several surgeons excised a fragment of their own skin (to show the patient that this was not painful) and then applied it to the patient's skin defect (Reverdin 1872). A study of publications on skin grafting at that time shows that virtually no author explained why homografts were used. Only occasionally is the remark found that the patients were afraid of pain at excision of skin fragments, or that additional scars at the donor site had to be avoided, especially in women (Lamm 1870; Heiberg 1871 a; Lesser 1873). On the other hand, friends and relatives were only too ready to contribute to healing by supplying fragments of skin (Bartlett 1872; Burdel 1875). Moreover, skin was easily obtained against some remuneration. Heiberg (1871 b) reported that the price of skin at the Berlin Military Hospital ranged from a groschen to a bottle of beer. The impression is sometimes created that homografts were used in particular for large skin defects such as burns (Clemens 1875) and abrasions (Brown 1879; Bradley 1881), because the patient himself was unable to supply enough skin, although only very small pieces of skin were used.

Sources of Skin for Homografting

All types of skin were initially considered suitable for grafting. The amount of skin which could be obtained from friends or relatives or from paid donors was

7 The reason why homografting was considered to be of equal value in the nineteenth century was in Gibson's opinion especially the result of the famous publication of Trembley (1744). Trembley performed homografting successfully in polyps (Gibson 1966).

limited. Soon therefore, efforts were made to find sources from which more skin could be obtained by a simple procedure. Amputated limbs were an obvious solution to the problem, for at that time amputations were among the most frequently performed operations. Amputations were done on patients with tuberculosis, non-specific bone infections, compound fractures, ulcers, tumours, and other lesions.

The surgeons in the major hospitals, where most of these amputations were performed, soon started to use skin from amputated limbs (Steele 1870; Cooper Forster 1871; Smith 1871; Anderson 1871; Hofmokl 1871; Heiberg 1871 a; Ollier 1872 a, b; Hickl 1875; Fischer 1880).

At smaller hospitals it was more difficult to obtain skin, but various ingenious ways to achieve that object were devised. One was to use the prepuce removed at circumcisions (Anger 1874; Lucas 1884).

In 1890, Ricketts still formally advocated the use of prepuce. Lucas (1884) a s urgeon in the Evelina Hospital for children, where circumcisions were regularly performed, described the use of perpuce in the treatment of a 30-month-old girl with abdominal burns. Prepuce was grafted onto the granulating surface (after cutting the prepuce into small fragments). The grafts "healed" quickly, and the girl was discharged from the hospital one month later. Lucas gave no further details.

Apart from the use of skin from live donors and from amputated limbs, the possibility of using skin from cadavers was investigated. In the *Centralblatt für Chirurgie* (1874), Menzel discussed an article by Porta (1874) in which the latter expressed his disappointment over his results with various skin grafts. Porta considered the use of cadaver skin as irresponsible. Menzel disagreed and wrote that he regarded cadaver skin as an important asset in skin grafting. By way of illustration he described how a patient with burns had benefited from cadaver skin grafts. After application of cadaver skin, the skin defects healed quickly. Menzel did not specify the thickness and size of the grafts, nor the duration of the follow-up. Years later, Girdner (1881) of New York again focused attention on the use of cadaver skin. In fact he claimed to have been the first to use cadaver skin. The case history presented by Girdner merits special mention.

A ten-year-old boy with burns of the left arm had skin defects which, once granulations had formed, were covered with cadaver skin. Four days later, 75% of the grafts had attached themselves to the underlying structure, and healing seemed to occur. Suddenly, something happened in the grafted area which Girdner described as follows: "... cicatrization would have doubtless gone on to a complete cure in a short time, but from an attack of erysipelatous inflammation a large portion of the newly formed skin was destroyed."

This could well have been erysipelas, as it was very common in the surgical wards at that time, on the other hand it could have been graft rejection.

Survival Chances of Homografts

The principal question raised in homografting was how long skin remained fit for use after excision. Some surgeons assumed that vitality was present as long as the skin was warm, and grafting could then be done. This conviction led to remarkable scenes. When Anger (1874) used skin from an amputated leg for grafting, he placed the patient whose leg was to be amputated and the patient who was to receive the grafts, side by side. After amputation followed excision and grafting of the skin. Jacenko (1871 b) thought of another way of keeping the graft warm. Whenever a leg was amputated somewhere in the hospital, the skin was immediately excised, and Jacenko placed the excised skin fragment in his armpit to keep it warm while he made his way to the patient who was to receive the graft!

Menzel (1872) who, like Jacenko, worked in Billroth's department in Vienna, reported that in 1872 virtually all grafts were performed with skin from amputated limbs but that, at that time, an interval of 90 minutes to eight hours between amputation and grafting was accepted. So different opinions existed about the question of whether grafts should be kept warm. He had read that Minich, in Venice, still obtained good results with cadaver skin excised nine hours after death. So far as could be established, Martin (1873) seems to have described the longest interval between amputation and excision of skin and grafting. Grafts excised from a leg amputated four days previously and stored at 10 °C, were successfully used, with favourable results (the term "favourable results" was not further qualified).

Complications in Homografting

Although homografts were as frequently used as autografts, cautions against their use gradually came to the fore because it was found that specific infections could be transmitted via homografts (Levis 1874). This was an important observation, because the skin used in homografting was often obtained from limbs which had been amputated for specific infections. Serious complications were described in several publications. One of the first was a report by Schaper (1872), describing transmission of smallpox.

An apparently healthy woman was admitted to the hospital where Schaper worked, after an accident in which her arm had been torn off. Skin was excised from this arm for grafting. The woman fell ill a few days later: she proved to have smallpox, and died. The skin from the arm had been used on four patients, three of whom developed smallpox. One died, and two recovered.

Shaper concluded that the smallpox must have been transmitted via the grafts. He advised that only skin from healthy individuals should be used for grafting, and that patients with pyaemia, syphilis, tuberculosis and smallpox should be excluded as donors.

Reverdin (1872) also cautioned explicitly against the use of skin from syphilitic patients. Deubel (1881) published the curious history of a case in which he believed that grafts had probably transmitted syphilis.

He had treated a patient with a large granulating perianal defect as a result of infected haemorrhoids. In three sessions this defect was covered with 85 grafts obtained from 12 donors. At the same time, 28 mucosal grafts obtained from rabbits were applied. One month after the first operation, an ulcer resembling a syphilitic ulcer developed in the grafted area. Subsequently, several more ulcers of the same appearance developed in this area. Ten weeks later the patient developed symptoms of secondary syphilis. At that time the patient's son reported to Deubel for medical treatment. It was found that he had contracted syphilis six months previously. The son had supplied several skin fragments for grafting! Deubel had no doubt that the father had contracted syphilis via the skin grafts from the son. Meanwhile, the patient's wife and a friend, who both nursed the patient, developed symptoms of syphilis. In Deubel's opinion they contracted syphilis through nursing the patient.

An example of possible transmission of tuberculosis via skin grafts was also found. Czerny (1886) described two patients in whom he considered it highly likely that their organ tuberculosis had been incurred via skin grafts. Both patients had burns, from which granulating defects had developed. These defects were covered with skin grafts obtained from a leg amputated for tuberculous arthritis. Although inoculation via the grafts could not be proven, Czerny expressed serious suspicions and advised that homografting be abandoned.

Unexplained Failures After Homografting

The first cautions against homografting came from surgeons who were afraid of transmitting (specific) infections. In addition, reports were published on unexplained local complications after homografting. The homografts had initially healed in the normal way, but ulceration had then developed in the grafted area for some obscure reason (Kappeler 1871; Jacenko 1871 b; Weiss 1872; Hewett 1875).

The descriptions seemed to indicate differences in the way in which such grafts degenerated. Kappeler described two patients whose skin grafts were at first accepted and increased in size, but subsequently diminished and finally disappeared completely. The duration of this process was not specified. Weiss expressed surprise at the fact that initial restoration of the circulation occurred in homografts, but that in a later stage a "fatal" blue colour developed beneath the grafts. While initially the grafts had seemed to be replaced by granulation tissue, an ulcer formed at the graft site. Jacenko using grafts with a diameter of 1–2 cm, observed that, initially, superficial erosions developed at the graft surfaces which gradually increased in size and depth and sometimes led to complete destruction of the grafts. At microscopic examination he saw a destructive process in the grafted area, and particularly in the Malpighian layer. Some of the large cells of this layer were filled with "pus corpuscles". One week after homografting, Hewett observed epithelialization along the edges of the grafts, while the centres were gradually absorbed. The absorption gradually spread until the grafts finally disappeared entirely. These authors all seem to describe a local rejection. However, it was to take years before the mechanism of this reaction was better understood. Even at this early stage, Weiss already advised on the basis of his experience with homografts that autografts were always to be preferred.

D. Heterografting

The applicability of heterografts was studied as intensively as that of homografts. Their clinical use was far less extensive.

Laboratory experiments were performed by such authors as Czerny (1871 b), Reverdin (1871 a, b) and Jacenko (1871 b). Some of Reverdin's experiments were performed in the laboratory of the celebrated French physiologist Claude Bernard in the *Collège de France* under supervision of Ranvier. Reverdin's reports on his experiments are somewhat confusing for us and hard to understand. He used rabbits, sheep and cats in reciprocal grafting experiments. Human skin was also grafted in these animals. Reverdin stated that all his experiments had been successful and that skin of one animal species could be grafted onto defects in the other species without problems. Jacenko (1871 b), too, maintained that human skin could be grafted onto animals. He had obtained favourable results with human skin grafts in dogs. Unfortunately, both investigators failed to specify the period covered by their observations, or the criteria of a "favourable result".

Besides these positive results, negative findings were also published, e.g. by Czerny (1871 b), who grafted human skin onto rats and dogs. He ascribed his poor results to the bad hygienic conditions in his laboratory. Probably Czerny was so intensively involved with heterografting because in his opinion the grafting activities in England and France went a lot further than in Germany and he was afraid that an important development would be missed. Clinical heterografting was done also, if to a more limited extent. Skin from several animal species was used. [8]

There was no consensus about the applicability of heterografts. Several authors were sceptical (Czerny 1871 b; Jacenko 1871 b; Weiss 1872; Darolles 1874). The grafts did attach themselves to the wound surface, and vascularization did subsequently occur, but after three to four weeks ulcers formed in the grafts and destroyed them (Weiss 1872; Darolles 1874). Porta (1874) who apparently had considerable experience with all kinds of skin grafting, reviewed his results after having performed 2516 grafts. He concluded that rabbit, dog, pigeon, and chicken skin grafts "nearly always" failed in human patients. He did add, however, that two grafts with dog skin had given satisfactory results (he, too, did not qualify the adjective "satisfactory").

A. Reverdin (1876) probably made the most persistent attempts to make heterografting a success.

He made these attempts in the case of a 21-year-old woman who had lost her entire scalp in an accident with a machine (see Fig. 11), and sought his advice six months after the accident. When healing ceased and no further cicatrization occurred, a large granulating defect remained. A. Reverdin treated one part of this defect with autografts, and used the other part for experiments with fragments of dog and rabbit skin; these grafts always disappeared after two or three days. After more than 50 unsuccessful attempts, Reverdin desisted and changed his experimental set-up. He assumed that granulation tissue played an important role in grafting and believed that better healing could be expected if he applied grafts whose undersurface was covered by granulation tissue. He obtained grafts with granulation tissue as follows: a U-shaped incision was made in the skin of the donor animal; the skin was carefully detached from the underlying structure, thus obtaining a kind of small pedicled full-thickness skin flap. Granulations formed on

---

8 Skin from dogs by Czerny (1871 b), Jacenko (1871 b), Netolitzky (1871), Dubrueil (1872), Porta (1874), Martin (1873), and Reverdin (1876). Rabbit skin by Netolitzky (1871), Reverdin (1871 a, b), Larrey (1872), Weiss (1872), Porta (1874), Darolles (1874), and Reverdin (1876). Rat skin by Czerny (1871 b), guinea-pig skin by Dubrueil (1872), sheep and cat skin by Reverdin (1871 a, b) and piglet skin by Raven (1877).

the undersurface of this flap within a few days, whereupon the pedicle was severed. The grafts were then placed on the granulating surface. Since these grafts, too, failed to attach themselves, the experiments were discontinued!

However, not only failures of heterografting were reported. J.-L. Reverdin (1871 a, b) reported on several successful grafts performed with animal skin. And so did Dubrueil (1872); he stated that, although the epidermis detached itself, the corium of the grafts remained vital. Neither Reverdin nor Dubrueil specified the duration of their follow-up. Raven (1877) did supply this information and this demonstrated the limited value of so-called "successful" grafts. He grafted piglet skin onto the skin defects in a patient with burns, and published the so-called "favourable" results of this operation within a few days. Beside the reports on successful heterografting in which the duration of the follow-up was unknown or very short, there were reports from surgeons who had not themselves observed the result.

The Russian surgeon Netolitzky (1871), who worked during the Franco-Prussian war as chief surgeon in a department for wounded soldiers in Bohemia, was asked to treat a 24-year-old woman who had lost her scalp in a accident, and still showed a skin defect two years later. Netolitzky applied autografts from the back of the hand, and heterografts obtained from a dog and a rabbit. He then continued his tour, and later he heard from a colleague that the grafts had been well accepted.

Larrey (1872) read a paper on behalf of Coze in which he discussed the good results obtained with rabbit skin grafts in three patients with an ulcer of the leg.

Apart from a few encouraging reports, little was heard about heterografting until 1884, when a paper by Allen (1884) attracted attention. Allen introduced frog

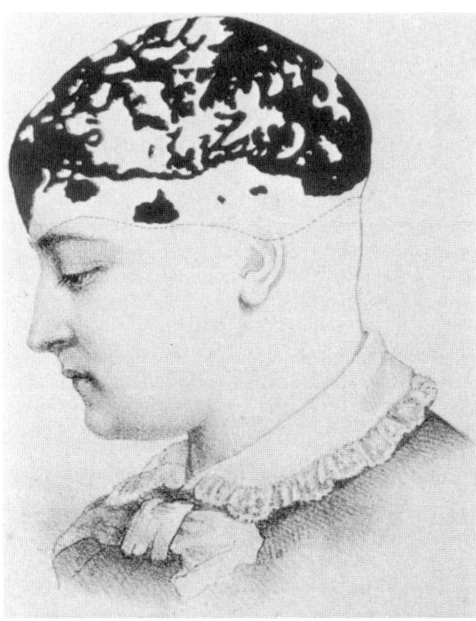

Fig. 11. A young woman who had lost her scalp in a machine accident. Reverdin (1876) performed several skin graft experiments on the granulating surface

skin as graft material. His idea was not really original, for Hanff (1870) had already used frog skin (see Chapt. 1).

Allen chose it because it has the same thickness throughout, was easily prepared and could be obtained from a virtually inexhaustible source (at least during the summer months). Allen did not specify what gave him the idea of using frog skin, but did give an account of the circumstances under which the operation was performed.

He wanted to perform a graft on a child with a granulating skin defect, but the parents refused to supply skin for their child. Allen then sent the child's father away with the assignment to catch frogs. The father subsequently brought several frogs to Allen's home. Allen stripped the skin off the frogs, wrapped it in gutta-percha tissue to prevent dehydration, took the parcels to the patient's home and there applied the frog skin to the skin defect.

When Allen published his results, he had treated three patients with frog skin. He reported that frog skin initially behaved like human skin, but later disappeared and was replaced by a thin transparent layer. Allen contended that epithelialization from the wound edges was stimulated by frog skin. The graft itself showed but little growth (what he meant by this is not clear from the text of his article).

Several doctors, e.g. Petersen (1885) of St. Petersburg, accepted Allen's suggestion and started grafting frog skin. Petersen wrote that the fragments of frog skin lost their colour after two or three days. He too, was impressed with the stimulating effects of frog skin on epithelization from the wound edges. Six weeks after application of the frog skin, the wound had healed with a firm, elastic scar.

Still no uniform criteria had been formulated on the basis of scientific facts with regard to indications for skin grafting, technique or type of transplant. That a uniform point of view was finally arrived at was thanks to Thiersch.

References

Abbe R (1878) Discussion: Entire scalp detached by machinery (Finell). Med Rec (1866–1922) 14:313

Allen W (1884) Skingrafts from the frog. Lancet 2:875

Anderson W (1871) Theory and practise of epidermic grafting. St Thom Hosp Rep 2:165–176

Anger B (1874) Sur l'hétéroplastie. CR Acad Sci (Paris) 79:1210–1212

Arnott H (1870) The treatment of ulcers and other granulating surfaces by transplantation of skin. Reports of hospital practise. Med Times Gaz 2:502

Ash V (1870) The rationale of skin-grafting (Letter to the editor). Lancet 2:913

Bardeleben A (1874) Lehrbuch der Chirurgie und Operationslehre. Reimer, Berlin

Barlow WH (1870) The operation of skin-grafting (Letter to the editor). Lancet 2:695

Bartlett SC (1872) Removal of entire scalp; wound healed by skingrafting. Am J Med Sci 64:573

Beigel H (1872) Transplantation kleiner Hautstücken zum Zwecke der Heilung torpider Geschwüre. Wien Med Wochenschr 22:573–577

Bellamy E (1870) The treatment of ulcers and other granulating surfaces by transplantation of skin. Reports of hospital practise. Med Times Gaz 2:503

Billroth Th (1866) Die allgemeine chirurgische Pathologie und Therapie. Reimer, Berlin

Billroth Th (1879) Chirurgische Klinik 1871–1876. Hirschwald, Berlin, p 461

Bligh JW (1873) Fenestrated non-adhesive plaster for skin-grafting (Letter to the editor). Lancet 1:360

Boeck (1872) Zur Lehre von der Hauttransplantation. Berl Klin Wochenschr 9:18

Bogg TW (1870) The rationale of skin-grafting (Letter to the editor). Lancet 2:913
Bradley WL (1881) Skin-grafting in loss of scalp. Med Rec (1866–1922) 19:231
Brown WS (1879) Skin-grafting. Boston Med Surg J 101:829–833
Bryant T (1871) Large ulcer on leg treated by skin-grafting. Med Times Gaz 2:188–189
Bryant T (1872) On skin-grafting. Guy's Hosp Rep 17:237–242
Burdel E (1875) Jeune fille entièrement scalpée par un arbre de couche en rotation. Union Med Prat Franc 19:458
Busch W (1872) Ueberpflanzung kleiner Hautstücken. Berl Klin Wochenschr 9:217
Chisolm JJ (1871) Skin-grafting. Med Rec (1866–1922) 5:534
Clemens FW (1875) Ueber Hauttransplantationen. Berl Klin Wochenschr 12:239
Coombs CP (1876) Cases of skin-grafting. Med Press 21:179
Cooper Forster (1871) Med Times Gaz 1:617
Coulson W (1871) Two patients with syphilitic ulcers cured by skin-grafting. Lancet 2:886–887
Couper J (1870) A case of skin-grafting on an ulcer of twenty-four years' standing. Lancet 2:602
Coupland (1874) Discussion: The mode of growth of new epithelium after skin-grafting (Golding Bird). Q J Micros Sci 14:421
Cowell G (1879) Case of complete removal of the scalp from injury. Lancet 2:421
Croft J (1870) Skin-grafting. Br Med J 2:616; Med Times 2:631
Czerny V (1870) Ueber Pfropfung von Epidermis auf granulirende Wundflächen. Zentralbl Med Wiss 8:881
Czerny V (1871 a) Ueber Pfropfung von Schleimhautepithel auf granulirende Wundflächen. Zentralbl Med Wiss 9:257
Czerny V (1871 b) Ueber Transplantationen. Wien Med Wochenschr 21:344
Czerny V (1886) Ueber die Entstehung der Tuberculose nach Hauttransplantationen. Verh Dtsch Ges Chir 15:22
Darolles MC (1874) Des greffes de lapin et de leur inutilité en chirurgie. Gaz Hebd Med Chir 11:400
Desprès (1869) Greffe épidermique (Reverdin). Bull Soc Chir Paris 10/2:511
Deubel (1881) Erysipèle gangréneux – emploi des greffes épidermiques pour hâter la cicatrisation. Inoculation de la syphilis par l'intermédiaire des greffes. Gaz Med Paris 3:628
Dobson NC (1870 a) The operation of skin-grafting (Letter to the editor). Lancet 2:695
Dobson NC (1870 b) A new method of treating ulcers by transplantation of skin. Med Times Gaz 2:500
Dobson NC (1870 c) The treatment of ulcers by transplantation of skin. Br Med J 2:563
Donnelly M (1872) Skin-grafting. Med Rec (1866–1922) 7:572–574
Dubrueil A (1872) Greffes animales transplantées sur l'homme. Bull Soc Chir Paris 1:365
Editorial (1870 a) The healing of wounds by transplantation. Lancet 2:62–63
Editorial (1870 b) Skin-grafting. Lancet 2:306–307
Editorial (1870 c) Skin-grafting. Br Med J 2:685
Ferguson J (1871 a) An instrument to facilitate skin-grafting. Lancet 1:745–746
Ferguson J (1871 b) Instrument for skin-grafting (Letter to the editor). Lancet 1:845
Fiddes D (1870) Skin-grafting (Letter to the editor). Lancet 2:870–871
Finnell (1878) Entire scalp detached by machinery – an immense granulating surface –. Med Rec (1866–1922) 14:313
Fischer E (1880) Ueber die künstliche Blutleere bei der Transplantation von Hautstücken. Dtsch Z Chir 13:193–195
Forster JC (1872) Clinical records. Guy's Hosp Rep 17:257 and 341
Freshwater F, Krizek TJ (1971) Skingrafting of burns: a centennial. J Trauma 11:862
Gibson T (1966) The first homografts: Trembley and the polyps. Br J Plast Surg 19:301
Gillespie (1871) Case of skin-grafting. Br Med J 1:60
Girdner JH (1881) Skingrafting with grafts taken from the dead subject. Med Rec (1866–1922) 20:119
Goldie RW (1871 a) On skin-grafting. Lancet 1:46

Goldie RW (1871 b) Epithelium and skingrafting. Lancet 1:534
Golding Bird CH (1874) The mode of growth of new epithelium after skin-grafting. Q J Micros Sci 14:420
Guipon (1874) Remarques à propos d'une nouvelle application des greffes épidermiques. Gaz Med Paris 252
Gussenbauer C (1883) Ueber Scalpirung durch Maschinengewalt. Z Heilk 4:380–392
Hamilton FH (1871) Healing of ulcers by transplantation. NY Med J 14:225–232
Hanff W (1870) Ueber Wiederanheilung vollständig vom Körper getrennter Hautstücke. Inaugural thesis. Lange Berlin Friedrich-Wilhelms-Universität
Haward JW (1871 a) Lancet 1:685, Med Times Gaz 1:617
Haward JW (1871 b) Sequel of Mr. Pollock's case of extensive burn healed by skin-grafting. Trans Clin Soc London 4:48–49
Haward JW (1871 c) Skin-grafting. Br Med J 1:568
Heath C (1870) The treatment of ulcers and other granulating surfaces by transplantation of skin. Reports of hospital practise. Med Times Gaz 2:502–503
Heiberg J, Schulz H (1871) Einiges über Hautverpflanzung. Berl Klin Wochenschr 8:112
Heiberg J (1871 a) Ueber die Bedeutung der Hauttransplantation. Berl Klin Wochenschr 8:612
Heiberg J (1871 b) Om Overplantning of Hudstykker. (Transplantation of skin) in Norwegian. Nor Mag Laegevidensk 1:167–170
Henne (1874) Drei Fälle von Hauttransplantation. Korrespondenzbl Schweiz Aerz 4: 289–293
Hewett P (1875) Old ulcer of leg; skingrafting; peculiar behaviour of engrafted skin. Lancet 1:124–125
Hickl (1875) Transplantation gänzlich abgetrennter Hautstücke. Wien Med Wochenschr 25:696
Hill B (1875) Skin-grafting upon a stump after amputation. Br Med J 2:719
Hodgen JT (1871) Cell or skingrafting. St Louis Med Surg J 8:289–294
Hofmokl (1871) Ueber einen Fall von Transplantation der Haut. Wien Med Wochenschr 21:292
Howard B (1871) Skin transplantation. Med Rec (1866–1922) 6:1830
Jacenko AS (1871 a) Kurze Mitteilung über Pfropfung der Haut auf Granulationsoberflächen. Berl Klin Wochenschr 8:85
Jacenko A (1871 b) Ueber die Transplantation abgetrennter Hautstücke. Med Jahrb 416–424
Johnson Smith (1870) The treatment of ulcers and other granulating surfaces by transplantation of skin. Reports of hospital practise. Med Times Gaz 2:504
Kappeler O (1871) Ueber die Inokulation und Transplantation kleiner Hautstücke auf Geschwüre und granulirende Wunden. Korrespondenzbl Schweiz Aerz 1:209–216
Kempe (1870) The treatment of ulcers and other granulating surfaces by transplantation of skin. Reports of hospital practise. Med Times Gaz 2:504
Knie A (1871) Ueber Wechseltransplantation. Zentralbl Med Wiss 9:819
Koch R (1878) Untersuchungen über die Aetiologie der Wundinfektionskrankheiten. Vogel Leipzig
Lamm A (1870) Om hudtransplantation såsom läkemetod för kroniska sår. (Skin grafting for treatment of ulcers) in Swedish. Hygiea (Stockh) 32:540–543
Larrey (1872) De l'emploi des greffes épidermiques pratiquées avec des lambeaux de peau de lapin pour la guérison des plaies rebelles. CR Acad Sci (Paris) 74:642
Lawson G (1870 a) Cases of skin-grafting. Lancet 2:567
Lawson G (1870 b) On the successful transplantation of portions of skin for the closure of large granulating surfaces. Med Times Gaz 2:631
Lawson G (1870 c) On the successful transplantation of portions of skin for the closure of large granulating surfaces. Lancet 2:708
Lawson G (1870 d) On the successful transplantation of portions of skin for the closure of large granulating surfaces. Br Med J 2:565
Lawson G (1871) On the transplantation of portions of skin for closure of large granulating surfaces. Trans Clin Soc London 4:49–53
Leale CA (1878) The use of common warts of the hand in skin-grafting. Med Rec (1866–1922) 14:188

Lesser (1873) Ueber Transplantation völlig getrennter Hautstücke auf Granulationsflächen. Berl Klin Wochenschr 10:62

Levis RJ (1874) Skin-grafting. Philad Med Times 4:389–391

Lindenbaum (1871) Ueber die Transplantation vollständig vom Körper getrennter Hautstücke auf granulirende Flächen. Berl Klin Wochenschr 8:128–132

Lindh A (1872) Några försök gjorda på Serafimerlasarettet, att öfverflytta hudstycken i sår. (Recent investigations on skin grafting in wounds) in Swedish. Hygiea (Stockh) 34: 69–74

Lloyd WmH (1876) Case of successful skin-grafting after amputation. Lancet 1:209

Lochner (1872) Zur Therapie der Fussgeschwüre. Arztl Intelligenzbl 19:388

Lucas RC (1884) On prepuce grafting. Lancet 2:586

Macleod GHB (1871 a) Skin-grafting (Letter to the editor). Lancet 1:806

Macleod GHB (1871 b) Remarks on skin-grafting. Br Med J 1:335–337

Macleod MD (1873) Mr J Bell's method of skin-grafting ulcers, with cases. Br Med J 2:84–85

Martin G (1873) De la greffe dans le traitement de l'ectropion. Ann Ocul 36/69:110–113

Mason F (1870 a) Cases of skingrafting. Lancet 2:566–567

Mason F (1870 b) The treatment of ulcers and other granulating surfaces by transplantation of skin. Reports of hospital practice. Med Times Gaz 2:502

Maurel E (1878) Note sur les greffes dermo-épidermiques dans différentes races humaines. Gaz Med Paris 7:349

Maxwell GT (1873) Grafting the skin of a white man upon a negro. Philad Med Times 4:37

McCarthy CW (1881) Observations on skin-grafting. Med Press 31:311–313

Menzel A (1872) Kleine Beiträge zur Hauttransplantation. Wien Med Wochenschr 22: 904–907

Mesterton CB (1871) Om öfverflyttning af hudstycken. (Skin transplantation) in Swedish Upsala Laekarefoeren Foerh 6:351–358

Morales R (1871) A successful case of transplantation. Med Rec (1866–1922) 6:80

Nehse H (1872) Ueber Transplantation. Inaugural thesis, Friedrich-Wilhelms-Universität Berlin, Schade, Berlin

Netolitzky J (1871) Zur Kasuistik der Hauttransplantation. Wien Med Wochenschr 21: 820–824

Nicholls J (1871) Skin-grafting. (Letter to the editor). Lancet 1:34

North A (1886) Covering the hand with skin transplanted from the chest. Med Rec (1866–1922) 29:36–39

Ollier LXEL (1872 a) Greffes cutanées ou autoplastiques. Bull Acad Méd (Paris) 1: 243–250

Ollier LXEL (1872 b) Des greffes cutanées. CR Acad Sci (Paris) 74:817–819

Paci A (1875) Osservazioni sul trapiantamento cutaneo. Sperimentale 36:36–61

Page D (1870) Observations on the true nature of the so-called "skin-grafting". Br Med J 2:655

Parish WH (1872) Skin-grafting as a treatment of indolent ulcers. Philad Med Times 3:168

Peet E (1977) Commentary. In: McDowell F The source book of plastic Surgery. Williams & Wilkins, Baltimore, p 30

Petersen O (1885) Ueber Transplantation von Froschhaut auf granulirende Wunden des Menschen. St Petersb Med Wochenschr (NF) 2:326

Pilcher JE (1881) Skin-grafting. Med Rec (1866–1922) 19:165

Pollock GD (1870 a) Skin-grafting and skin-transplantation. Br Med J 2:565

Pollock GD (1870 b) Skin-grafting and skin-transplantation. Med Times Gaz 2:630

Pollock GD (1870 c) Mr. Pollock's case of skin transplantation. Lancet 2:686

Pollock GD (1870 d) The operation of skin-transplantation; clinical remarks. Lancet 2: 669–670

Pollock GD (1870 e) Several cases of skin-grafting and skin-transplantation. Lancet 2: 707

Pollock GD (1870 f) Skin-grafting. Lancet 1:680

Pollock GD (1871) Cases of skin-grafting and skin-transplantation. Trans Clin Soc London 4:37–49

Pollock GD (1873) Skin-grafting. Lancet 1:680

Poncet A (1871) Des greffes dermo-épidermiques et en particulier des larges lambeaux dermo-épidermiques. Lyon Med 8:494, 520, 564
Pooley JH (1871) Report of the surgical cases treated in the St. John's Riverside Hospital. NY Med J 21:490
Porta L (1874) Ueber Epidermis-Pfropfung auf Wunden (Report by Menzel). Zentralbl Chir 1:168
Ranke H (1871) Ueber Reverdin's Verfahren der Verpflanzung von Hauttheilchen auf granulirende Wundflächen behufs Beschleunigung der Vernarbung. Aerztl Intelligenzbl 18:80
de Ranse F (1870) Greffe épidermique. Gaz Med Paris 343
Raven TF (1877) Skin-grafting from the pig. Br Med J 2:623
Reverdin A (1876) Ein Fall von Abreissung der Kopfhaut, durch Transplantationen geheilt. Dtsch Z Chir 6:418
Reverdin H (1971) Jaques-Louis Reverdin. Sauerländer, Aarau
Reverdin JL (1869) Greffe épidermique. Bull Soc Chir Paris 10:511–515
Reverdin JL (1871 a) Sur la greffe épidermique. CR Acad Sci (Paris) 73:1280–1282
Reverdin JL (1871 b) Greffe épidermique. CR Soc Biol (Paris) 23:147
Reverdin JL (1872) De la greffe épidermique. Arch Gen Med [Suppl 6] 19:276, 555, 703
Ricketts BM (1890) Some observations on bone and skingrafting. Med Rec (1866–1922) 38:504
Rodriguez EF (1871) Transplantation in a case of serpiginous phagedaena. Med Rec (1866–1922) 6:463
Schaper (1872) Uebertragung der Pocken durch Implantation während des Prodromalstadiums. Dtsch Militairärztl Z 1:53
Schede (1881) Die Reverdin'schen Transplantation. Dtsch Med Wochenschr 7:352
Schweniger E (1875) Ueber Transplantation und Implantation von Haaren. Z Biol (Munich) 11:341
Sée M (1870) Epidermic grafting. Med Times Gaz 2:42–43
Smith (1871) On skin grafting. Med Times Gaz 1:617
Steele C (1870) Transplantation of skin. Br Med J 2:621
Storch O (1871) Jagttagelser over Hudpodning. (On skin transplantation) in Norwegian. Ugeskr Laeg 11:169
Studensky N (1873) Zur Frage über die Hauttransplantation auf Geschwüre. Zentralbl Med Wiss 11:193–195
Tait L (1870) The treatment of ulcers and other granulating surfaces by transplantation of skin reports of hospital practise. Med Times Gaz 2:502
Thierfelder A (1872) Ueber Anheilung transplantirter Hautstücke. Arch Heilk 13:524–531
Thiersch C (1874) Ueber die feineren anatomischen Veränderungen bei Aufheilung von Haut auf Granulationen. Langenbecks Arch Chir 17:318; Verh Dtsch Ges Chir 3:69–75
Trembley A (1744) Mémoires, pour servir à l'histoire d'un genre de polypes d'eau douce, à bras en forme de Cornes. Verbeek, Leide
Trueheart CW (1871) Discussion: the treatment of cicatricial contractions after burns of the face (Buck). Med Rec (1866–1922) 6:212
Watson WS (1871) Unsuccessful skin-grafting for protracted ulceration of a burn in the dorsal and lumbar regions – death under influence of chloroform. Br Med J 1:641
Weiss C (1872) Ueber Transplantation gänzlich abgetrennter Hautstücke. Inaugural thesis, Fues, Universität Tübingen
Wierx van Rhijn EMF (1874) Iets over huidtransplantatie. (On Skin transplantation) in Dutch. Thesis, University Utrecht Kemink en Zoon, Utrecht
Wilson JM (1870) Skin-grafting. Br Med J 2:694
Wolfe JR (1875) A new method of performing plastic operations. Br Med J 2:360–361
Wood MA (1871) Skin-grafting under ether-spray. Br Med J 1:446–447
Woodman J (1871) Notes on transplantation or engrafting of skin. Churchill, London
Woodman J (1873) Skin-grafting. Br Med J 2:114
Wurfbain CL (1871) Huid-transplantatie. (Skin transplantation) in Dutch. Werk Genootsch Bevord Nat-Genees-Heelk [Amst] 2:12

Chapter 3
Skin Grafting in Eyelid Surgery

After its initial heyday (1869–1874), skin grafting to accelerate wound healing entered a period of decline, until its use almost ceased. While skin grafts were used only very sparingly in general surgery between 1874 and 1886, they were frequently used during these years in a particular branch of surgery: palpebral surgery. The grafts used in palpebral surgery were mostly full-thickness skin grafts. One of the reasons for their successful use in this branch of surgery must have been that the defects to be covered were smaller than those in general surgery. The wound beds in most of these cases were well vascularized. Little is known about this aspect of skin grafting in the surgical world, probably because reports were mostly published in ophthalmological journals. The main purpose of skin grafting as advocated by Reverdin was to accelerate the healing of skin defects. It was soon understood that skin grafts could also be used for other purposes. Particularly surgeons who treated patients with insufficiencies of palpebral skin, leading to ectropion which in turn led to corneal abnormalities, soon discovered the value of grafts to cover these defects.

A. Lawson's Successful Reconstruction

The British surgeon Lawson (1870a, b, 1871; Fig. 12) was probably the first to perform a successful reconstruction of an eyelid with the aid of skin grafts. On 14th October 1870, Lawson admitted to the Royal London Ophthalmic Hospital a patient with complete ectropion of the upper eyelid, which had developed as a result of lupus vulgaris. The next day, he performed an operation on this patient. The cicatricial tissue was incised and excised, and this made it possible to establish contact between upper and lower eyelids. The margins of the palpebrae were then sutured together with two stitches, thus obtaining a surface of fixed dimensions. Three days later, granulation tissue had developed in the defect, and a skin graft the size of a "silver threepenny coin", diameter 16 mm (Fig. 13), was applied; it had been obtained from the inside of the patient's upper arm and the subcutaneous fat had been removed before the graft was applied.

The eyelid with the graft was covered with an isinglass plaster, on top of which a cotton wool compress was placed, and then a dressing to ensure fixation. The unaffected eye was likewise covered with a cotton wool dressing. Two days later, a

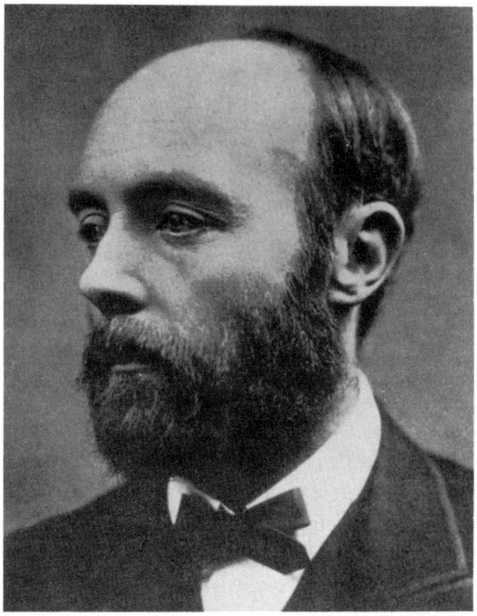

Fig. 12. George Lawson (1831 – 1903) who probably performed the first well-documentated successful full-thickness skin graft in the reconstruction of an upper eyelid (McDowell 1977)

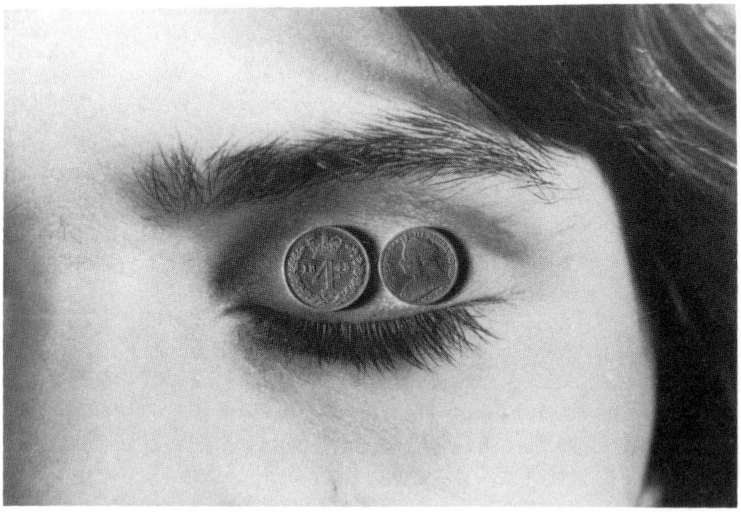

Fig. 13. Lawson used full thickness skin grafts as large as a silver threepenny, respectively silver fourpenny piece

full-thickness skin graft the size of a "silver fourpenny coin", diameter 17 mm, was applied to another part of the granulating surface.

The two grafts were accepted and 14 days after the first operation the entire defect was "skinned over" (covered by epithelium). Lawson stated that sensibility had also been recovered during this period, because the patient felt the grafts being touched with a blunt object.

Lawson concluded that full-thickness grafts on granulating defects of the eyelids were able to heal, provided they were carefully applied and firmly fixed in position. A dressing was considered useful to keep the grafts at body temperature.

The technique described by Lawson was used for many years, virtually unchanged. Although the operation seemed successful according to the description, the question remained why Lawson never again mentioned this technique; and specifically not in his books, e.g. in the second edition of *Diseases and Injuries of the Eye,* which appeared in 1874 (first edition: 1869) (Lawson 1874). Wolfe later used this fact as an argument in support of his assumption that something might have gone wrong after the operation and that consequently he (Wolfe) was the first to perform the operation successfully.

B. Other Initiatives in Eyelid Grafting

Not only in Great Britain but in other parts of the world as well, surgeons practising palpebral surgery wondered whether skin grafts could be used in the treatment of anomalies of the eyelids. At the annual meeting of the *Ophthalmologische Gesellschaft* in Heidelberg, Strube (1871) of Bremen started a discussion of the value of skin grafts in the treatment of palpebral skin defects, e.g. as a result of burns. Horner (1871) of Zürich responded with the remark that all surgeons treating patients with burns of the eyelids should use skin grafts. Only thus could a soft scar of the eyelid be obtained, with less contraction of the adjacent tissues. Driver (1871) in the same session presented a patient who had developed ectropion of the lower eyelids after sustaining burns of the cheek. The cicatricial tissue which had caused the ectropion was excised and the two eyelids were sutured together with a few stitches; the defect was covered with grafts obtained from the patient's upper eyelid and upper arm. Driver probably used full-thickness grafts; there were six, each the size of a lentil. Three of the grafts were accepted and attached themselves to the wound surface. The operation was performed a few weeks before the meeting at which Driver reported the case. His description gives the impression that the grafts were applied to the fresh wound floor, although he did not state this explicitly.

Another early report came from the United States: Hamilton (1871), a celebrated surgeon, working at that time in New York, also used skin grafts in the reconstruction of an eyelid with ectropion. He applied them to the granulating surface obtained after excision of the cicatricial tissue. Unfortunately, Hamilton did not specify how long it was after grafting before he concluded that the operation had been successful.

It was soon established by Menzel (1872) that early acceptance of the grafts was hardly predictive of the ultimate result. In the reconstruction of an eyelid, nine small skin grafts were applied to the skin defect, and accepted; ultimately so much contraction occurred that the result did not differ from the preoperative situation. It is to be noted that in the patient described by Menzel, the skin defects mostly healed by epithelialization from the grafts.

In France, too, attention was focused on the use of skin grafts in eyelid reconstruction. Although autografts were used nearly everywhere, Le Fort (1872) opted in favour of a homograft. According to him homografts gave equally good results. He described the operative treatment of a patient with a skin defect of one eyelid, with the aid of a full-thickness skin homograft, and reported a perfect and lasting cure. The large graft was subsequently identifiable only by its colour, which differed from that of adjacent parts. He advocated the use of a single large graft instead of several small ones in palpebral reconstruction, because this should ensure that contraction did not occur. The use of skin grafts in palpebral surgery in France was stimulated in particular by de Wecker and his co-workers (de Wecker 1872, 1873; Martin 1873; Masselon 1875).

De Wecker wondered why skin grafting had failed to assume the same importance in palpebral surgery as in general surgery. When he started using grafts, he introduced what he called "mosaic grafting": full-thickness pieces of skin with a diameter of 0.6–0.8 cm were applied to the defect in a mosaic pattern. In operations for correction of ectropion, 20–30 such grafts were used. Autografts as well as homografts were used (Masselon 1875). In the hospital where these operations were performed, there was in fact a lively trade in skin. The price ultimately rose to 10 francs per square centimetre!

Not only was skin from paid donors used, but also skin obtained from patients with entropion or trichiasis, treated by excision of a strip of skin. And skin from amputated limbs was also used. In patients with burns of the eyelids, skin grafting was done as soon as the necrotic tissue was shed and granulation tissue formed; this was done to prevent ectropion so far as possible (Martin 1873). Grafting was done also when ectropion had already occurred as a result of burns; also in ectropion due to other causes, e.g. lupus vulgaris, and in skin defects caused by excision of tumours.

Initially, many small grafts were used in the treatment of patients with fresh wounds, but the policy was later changed in favour of the use of a single large graft, which was sutured in position (Masselon 1875).

Another French surgeon, Sichel (1875), likewise reported successful palpebral reconstruction. In one of his patients, with ectropion of the upper eyelid as a result of burns, two previous attempts at reconstruction had failed. In the third attempt, a piece of skin measuring 5×4 cm was excised from the patient's upper arm. The subcutaneous tissue was removed, and the skin was cut into smaller fragments, which were grafted onto the defect resulting from excision of the cicatrical tissue. This defect measured 4.5×2.5 cm. The grafts were readily accepted, and nine days after the operation the case was presented to the members of the *Société de Chirurgie de Paris* as an example of a successful graft.

C. Wolfe and the Full-Thickness Skin Graft

In the same year, Wolfe's reconstruction of an eyelid attracted most attention (Wolfe 1875). In fact admiration for Wolfe, who used full-thickness skin grafts, was so great that his name was attached to these grafts in English-speaking countries (Wolfe grafts).

Wolfe (1824–1904), surgeon to the Glasgow Ophthalmic Institution, presented his technique in the *British Medical Journal* as a novelty. He had begun to use free skin grafts because he believed that the pedicle of pedicled flaps made no contribution whatsoever to the vitality of the flap! The patient on whom he performed the reconstruction had sustained injuries of both eyes in a gunpowder explosion. Wolfe described the correction of one of the lower eyelids. The upper eyelid of the same eye had previously been corrected with the aid of skin grafts, but he supplied no data on this previous operation. The cicatricial tissue of the everted lower eyelid was excised; the edges of the two eyelids were sutured together, resulting in a skin defect measuring 5×3.5 cm. Three pieces of skin were excised from the patient's forearm. The subcutaneous tissue of two was removed

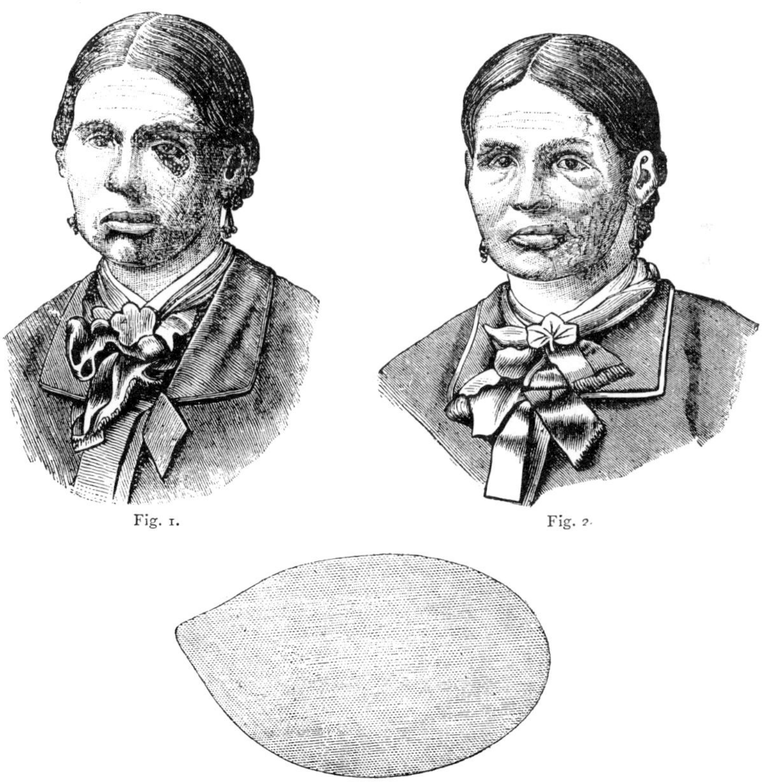

Fig. 14. An artists' impression of the face of a woman before and after reconstruction of an eyelid in which a full thickness skin graft was used (Wolfe 1881)

until the undersurface assumed a whitish colour. The subcutaneous tissue of the third graft was removed less carefully. The three grafts were applied to the skin defect. The two grafts whose subcutaneous tissue had been carefully removed healed. The graft from which the subcutaneous tissue had been less carefully removed started suppurating after four days; only a small part of this graft remained intact. The sutures keeping the eyelids together were removed on the fourth postoperative day. Wolfe did not specify the duration of his follow-up in his publication. After reporting in the *British Medical Journal* he asserted himself as a fervent advocate of full-thickness skin grafts, and stressed the fact that he had been the first to use this technique.

He did this mostly in letters to the editors of various journals. In 1880 he sent a letter to the editor of the *Zentralblatt für praktische Augenheilkunde,* in which he commented on a publication in which the well-known German ophthalmic surgeon Zehender (1879) in Rostock had reported several failures with full-thickness skin grafts in palpebral reconstruction (Wolfe 1880). Wolfe held that Zehender had made several technical mistakes; for example, he had used sutures to keep the grafts in position. Wolfe described this as a serious flaw – a strange remark in view of the fact that another of Wolfe's publications (1881) shows that he himself used sutures for graft fixation: "It (the graft) was then applied to the gap in the eyelid, to which it was united by fine silk ligatures" (Fig. 14).

From his letter to the editors of the *Zentralblatt für praktische Augenheilkunde* it appears that Wolfe's statements have to be regarded with a certain amount of reserve. With reference to a remark that skin grafting could not always be successful in palpebral surgery, he mentioned having treated a 60-year-old man with ectropion of the upper and lower eyelids of one eye. Of the attempts to reconstruct both eyelids, one failed and the other was entirely successful. In the latter case, however, skin from a son of the patient had been used!

Wolfe's self-assertion was not always applauded, as the following anecdote demonstrates. An anonymous reporter stated in the *Lancet* in 1882 that a patient was treated with everted upper and lower eyelids. Reconstruction was effected with the aid of full-thickness skin grafts. It was noted in the article that the operation was performed by *the method which Lawson had described in 1870,* although a single large graft was used for each eyelid and was applied to the fresh wound surface. Wolfe (1882) immediately sent a letter to the editor of the *Lancet.* He stated that *he* had introduced this operation and that *his* operation differed from Lawson's "in principle and practise". The editors coolly replied that they had been unable to discover any difference "in principle and practise" between Lawson's method and Wolfe's. Lawson himself ignored Wolfe's letter completely.

D. Further Application of the Full-Thickness Skin Graft

Another report on full-thickness skin grafting of the upper eyelid, or in other words a report on replantation or reimplantation was found in the British literature of 1875. Taylor (1875) operated on a patient with ptosis which he wanted to correct by excising part of the upper eyelid. After excising the skin and closing the wound, Taylor found that the patient could no longer close the eye. He therefore restored the excised skin to its original position and fixed it with sutures. The skin was completely accepted.

Interest in full-thickness skin grafts had been aroused, and in several countries such grafts were used in the treatment of various abnormalities of the eyelids, usually in the patients with ectropion as a result of burns. The reports on this operation as a rule concerned a single patient. The results varied. Poor results were due to disturbed graft acceptance or subsequent graft contraction.

Particularly in the 1880s this subject received much attention. In France, most patients were presented at meetings of the *Société de Chirurgie de Paris* (Meyer 1881; Berger 1881, 1888; Monod 1881), and the problems of acceptance and contraction were predominant at these meetings. Berger (1881) described the problems of graft acceptance he had encountered in a patient with ectropion, whose skin defect had been covered with a graft. The graft, taken from the patient's back, was only partly accepted. The remainder of the skin defect healed by secondary epithelialization which caused contraction. In 1888 Berger presented another case in which an analogous procedure had been followed. The graft had healed, but severe contraction had occurred. In the discussion after this presentation a member of the audience remarked that the skin of the back was unsuitable for palpebral grafting. It was considered advisable to use skin which had approximately the same properties as the eyelid skin. Meyer also described ultimate contraction of a skin graft placed on the lower eyelid after excision of a tumor. The graft healed but its diameter diminished by 50% within a month.

The results described in the British literature in that decade did not differ too much from the French results. Snell (1882) and Streatfield (1884) achieved only partial improvement of ectropion with their reconstructions. Snell operated on a patient with a chronic fistulous process near the eyelids, and Streatfield on a patient with congenital syphilis.

Hume (1882) likewise observed several failures, but was successful in one patient with an upper eyelid everted as a result of burns. Toswill (1882) also described a good result, in a boy with burn scars of both eyelids which were reconstructed in one session. Not only were the grafts accepted but not a trace of contraction was observed four months after the operation. The grafts differed from adjacent tissue only in colour. McHardy (1881) was one of the few who could present a case with a longer follow-up than one year.

The Americans did not lag behind. Wadsworth (1876) was one of the first American surgeons to reconstruct eyelids with the aid of skin grafts. Wolfe had already mentioned him several times as one of the first surgeons to adopt his technique. Wadsworth performed his reconstructions with the aid of a single skin graft which was nearly twice the size of the skin defect.

Other Americans, e.g. Aub (1879), form Cincinnati, agreed with Wadsworth that the grafts should be twice as large as the defects to be repaired. He reached his conclusion, independent of Wadsworth, on the basis of personal observation indicating that, after healing, the grafts gradually diminished in size by about 40%. Once Aub started using larger skin grafts, his results improved. Aub's statements carried weight, for he evaluated his results two years after the operation. In the

United States, too, surgeons struggled with the same problems as their colleagues elsewhere in the world: disturbed graft healing and contraction.

Mathewson (1880), Kipp (1880) and Noyes (1880) described several cases in which grafts failed to heal; in the cases in which healing did occur, considerable contraction developed. Kipp (1880) reported failure of grafting in two of the four patients. In the other two, the result initially seemed good, but subsequent contraction led to the same situation as that which prevailed prior to the operation.

Howe (1880) initially seemed to obtain a good result, but the diameter of the graft diminished by 25% within two months. Noyes (1880) observed the same phenomenon: the grafts failed to heal in two of his three patients. In the third patient – a boy with ectropion of both upper eyelids as a result of burns – the skin defect of one of the eyelids was covered with a full-thickness skin graft almost twice the size of the defect. The graft was obtained from the chest wall, and was washed with warm water to keep it at the right temperature until application. Seven weeks later, after undisturbed healing, the size of the graft had diminished by 25%. Hardly any sensibility had been recovered, and the colour of the graft differed markedly from that of adjacent tissues.

Skin grafts were used, not only to repair defects of the eyelid skin but also to repair conjunctival defects. Ely (1881) presented an example of this application. A 50-year-old man had sustained facial burns in a gunpowder explosion. He had lost his right eye, and the burn scar had completely obliterated the cul-de-sac of the left eye. An attempt was made to reconstruct the cul-de-sac. The eyelid was detached from the eyeball, and a skin graft was applied to the fresh wound surface on the inside of the eyelid and sutured in position with a few stitches. The graft was accepted, but contraction occurred at the conjunctival fold, thus reducing the depth of the cul-de-sac. Ely was nevertheless satisfied with the result, particularly because, as he said, no antiseptic precautions had been taken during the operation, and the graft had been handled fairly roughly; during excision of the subcutaneous fat, it had twice been dropped on the floor! Ely did not say why he attached such importance to antiseptic precautions. The fact that the graft was accepted had probably exceeded his expectations.

In German-speaking countries, too, several publications reported on the use of full-thickness skin grafts in reconstruction of eyelids. Here, too, appreciation of this technique varied. Zehender (1879) and the Polish surgeon Wicherkiewicz (1882) obtained mainly poor results. Beside his poor results, the latter described some successes which the modern reader cannot fail to query. For example, he described a good result in a patient whose ectropion was corrected with the aid of a homograft. He concluded that results could probably be improved by two measures. To begin with, by antiseptic precautions to reduce the risk of infection and ensure better healing. He preferred a 5% carbolic acid (phenol) solution as an antiseptic. Secondly, bleeding of the wound bed had to be arrested before application of the graft, because blood between wound bed and graft prevented acceptance of the graft. Wicherkiewicz decided that in future he would apply skin grafts only to granulating surfaces.

Kuhnt (1883) a pupil of Becker and working in Jena devised a very different approach to the problem of preventing blood accumulation beneath the graft. To ensure adequate drainage, he made several incisions in the grafts. This was also advised by Fischer (1880) and later by Vogel (1907) and Försterling (1907). In recent literature they are honoured for having been the first to introduce this solution (Zoltan 1962).

Beside the poor results reported by Zehender and Wicherkiewicz, good results were described by Schede (1881), Samelsohn (1881), Kuhnt (1883) and Bock (1884). It is questionable whether Samelsohn's name should be mentioned in this context, for in fact he did not use a free skin graft but a pedicled flap from the temporal region and repaired the defect of the temporal region with a skin graft. Schede (1881) achieved adequate drainage of the wound surface by applying many small ellipsoid grafts (maximum length 1.5 cm) to the surface in a mosaic pattern.

One of the largest series of eyelid reconstructions was presented by Bock (1884), who described the results obtained in Stellwag von Carion's department in Vienna. Skin grafting of the eyelids was performed for several different reasons on no fewer than 18 patients. The results were evaluated as good in the majority of these cases. It is to be noted that the sole criterion of a "good" result was the acceptance of the graft. The result was always evaluated at the patient's discharge from the hospital. In Stellwag von Carion's department, too, several small grafts were applied to the defect instead of a single large one. This facilitated application of the grafts and ensured better adhesion. If one or several small grafts failed to heal, they could be removed and replaced by other grafts. Bock did not mention the advantage of adequate drainage. Autografts were used in all patients except one, who received a homograft.

E. The Split-Skin Graft in Eyelid Surgery

After Thiersch (1886) had read his paper advocating the use of split-skin grafts, these grafts were also used again in surgery of the eyelids, especially since several surgeons believed that these grafts did not contract (Everbusch 1887a; Laqueur 1887). Everbusch in fact used very thin grafts which consisted only of epidermis and the top surface of the papillary layer. In Thiersch's department, favourable results were obtained with split-skin grafts in reconstruction of eyelids (Plessing 1888; Urban 1892).

F. Dressing Technique

Several different types of dressing were used. In many cases the grafts were first covered with a non-adhesive layer to prevent their removal at a change of dressing. Well-known examples were goldbeater's skin (Sichel 1875; Noyes 1880) and silver foil (Bock 1884). Others tried to prevent adhesion to the dressing by greasing the latter; Lawson (1882), for example, used greased lint. Hume (1882) and Wicherkiewicz (1882) moistened the dressing with warm water for this reason. There was no pronounced preference for a single layer or several layers of dressing. The dressing used by Kuhnt (1883) illustrates how complex the dressing technique could be. After grafting, he painted the wound with iodoform and covered it with silk taffeta or goldbeater's skin; this was covered with a layer of iodoform gauze, followed by a layer of cotton wool soaked in a 10% carbolic acid (phenol) solution; finally, a bandage was applied to keep everything in position. The first change of dressing was usually not made until the third day (Monod 1881).

G. Results

Several articles were published which reviewed the results obtained in reconstructive palpebral surgery (Monod 1881; Bouvin 1883). The conclusions did not differ too much. It was advised that only autografts be used (Lucas Championnière 1888). The subcutaneous tissue of full-thickness grafts had to be carefully removed before use. Most surgeons preferred a single large graft to several small ones. The grafts were preferably sutured in position (Howe 1880; Snell 1882; Toswill 1882), but there was no consensus on this point; in some cases, sutures were deliberately avoided so as not to damage the grafts (Noyes 1880; Berger 1881). The use of antisepsis remained another debatable point. Some surgeons regarded antisepsis as an absolute prerequisite to success (Wicherkiewicz 1882), whereas others thought it quite unimportant (Bock 1884). The ophthalmic surgeon Bouvin in the Hague expressed in 1883 the wish that the results of palpebral reconstruction should not be published until a year after the operation, because healing of the graft determined only part of the ultimate result. He regarded the contraction (which occurred at a much later stage) as a serious complication. To prevent contraction, the use of grafts at least twice as large as the defect was advocated (Berger 1881; Monod 1881; Kuhnt 1883; Silex 1896).

H. Skin Grafting in Other Eyelid Abnormalities

Not only in the case of ectropion were skin grafts used for reconstruction, although ectropion as a result of burns was the principal indication. One of the reasons for using skin grafts especially in this type of ectropion was that burns caused lesions which were not confined to the eyelids but also involved adjacent tissues. This made it difficult to use pedicled flaps.

Gradually, skin grafts were being used more and more in the treatment of other abnormalities of the eyelids as well. The discussion which followed a paper which Vossius (1887) read at the annual meeting of the *Ophthalmologische Gesellschaft* in Heidelberg, on the operative treatment of trichiasis, showed that skin grafts were often used in these cases also by other ophthalmic surgeons, such as Wicherkiewicz (1887), Everbusch (1887 b) and von Hippel (1887). In this operation, the zone between the anterior and the posterior palpebral limbus was incised over the entire length of the eyelid. The resulting defect was closed with the aid of a full-thickness skin graft (Wicherkiewicz 1887; von Hippel 1887 and Raehlmann 1891), or a split-skin graft (Jaesche 1881; Everbusch 1887 b; Franke 1890). Hotz (1892) made experiments to establish whether, in patients with a large pterygium, he could use skin grafts to prevent the relapses otherwise regularly observed after excision. After excision of the pterygium, the defect in the conjunctiva of the eyeball was closed with a thin skin graft. He was highly satisfied with the results. No relapse had occurred a few months after the operation. The grafts assumed a smooth, transparent appearance and hardly protruded from the conjunctiva of the eyeball.

J. Skin Grafting on Fresh Eyelid Wounds

Publications on skin grafting on fresh palpebral wounds were scanty (Horner 1871; Martin 1873). Most ophthalmic surgeons confronted with fresh wounds waited until granulation tissue developed. Few attempted early grafting. In this respect, Raehlmann (1891) and Pfalz (1905, 1908) did pioneering work. Raehlmann advised grafting at an early stage, but supplied no specific data on the time of operation. He described a patient who sustained palpebral burns on Christmas Eve: grafting was done six days later.

Pfalz (1908) supplied more details in an article entitled "Ueber Frühtransplantation bei Verbrennungen der Augenlider". [1] Pfalz worked in the Ruhr area, where accidents with molten steel regularly occurred in the steel mills. Hot steel droplets often caused eyelid burns. Initially, Pfalz believed that conservative treatment of these lesions led to a fair cure. It was later found that healing was followed a few months later by contraction which gave rise to a variety of complications, ectropion, entropion, trichiasis, epiphora and symblepharon. He sought a method to prevent these complications and found that much better results were obtained when the grafts were applied at an early stage. Initially, he did operate earlier, but still waited until spontaneous demarcation of the necrotic tissue occurred (Pfalz 1905); later he no longer waited for this, but removed the necrotic tissue mechanically. Granulation tissue was thus prevented from developing. The time of operation was determined by the depth of the burns. In the case of superficial burns the necrotic tissue was removed on the third or fourth day; in the case of deeper burns it was done on the sixth or seventh day. Pfalz unfortunately did not mention by what criteria he distinguished between superficial and deep burns.

Grafts were used also on small burns; Pfalz indicated that excision and grafting should be done when the burns were the size of a pea. When the burns were localized near the medial canthus or the lacrimal sac, excision and grafting were resorted to even if the burns were only lentil-sized. The necrotic tissue was removed with a curette until a bleeding surface was obtained. A razor was then used to cut the thinnest possible graft, which was applied to the fresh wound surface as soon as bleeding ceased. Pfalz took no special measures to ensure fixation of the grafts. They were merely covered with wet gauze. When the graft had failed to attach itself to the surface after 48 hours, it was removed and a new graft was applied one day later.

---

1 Early skin grafting in burns of the eyelids.

The operative treatment was not confined to the outer palpebral surface but also included conjunctival lesions. All burns on the conjunctival surface of the eyelid were grafted if they extended beyond half the height of the conjunctiva or covered more than a quarter of its width. Pfalz knew from experience that conservative treatment was followed by contraction which gave rise to serious complications. He saw mostly burns of the upper eyelids; when burns involved the conjunctival surface, the lower eyelid was usually also damaged.

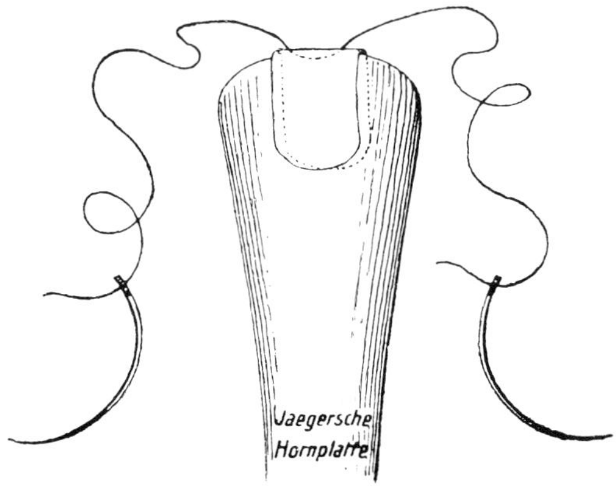

Fig. 15. The horn plate, a useful aid in the application of skin grafts on the conjunctival side of the eyelids (Pfalz 1908)

Initially, Pfalz covered defects resulting from conjunctival burns with mucosal grafts obtained from the buccal surface of the cheek or from the lip. Mucosal tissue showed a marked tendency to contract, and the technique was difficult. He obtained much better results with thin skin grafts instead of mucosal grafts. Pfalz called these grafts epidermal grafts. They could be applied to the wound bed without much difficulty, and gave good functional results. Contraction scarcely occurred. He did observe that the skin grafts never merged into mucosal tissue. Pfalz placed the skin grafts in position with a simple instrument which look ed like a shoehorn (Fig. 15). The graft was folded over the "shoehorn" with the under-surface up, and then inserted between eyelid and eyeball. It was fixed in position with transcutaneous sutures. Pfalz concluded that early excision and grafting could prevent complications such as contraction! It appears that Pfalz was the first to perform early excision and grafting on a large scale. It is remarkable that his publication never received the attention it deserved. Yet the therapeutic principles formulated by Pfalz are still valid today.

References

Aub J (1879) Ectropium durch Transplantation von Hautstücken ohne Stiel (Pedicle) behandelt. Arch Augenheilkd 8:400–408

Berger P (1881) Ectropion considérable de la paupière inférieure. Greffe par transplantation d'un lambeau taillé par de peau du dos, combinée avec la blepharorraphie. Bull Soc Chir Paris 7:678

Berger P (1888) Greffes cutanées. Bull Soc Chir Paris 14:48
Bock E (1884) Die Pfropfung von Haut und Schleimhaut auf oculistischen Gebiete. Braumüller, Wien
Bouvin MJ (1883) Plastische operaties der oogleden met ongesteelde huidlappen. (Free skin grafts around the eye) in Dutch. Ned. Tijdschr Geneeskd 20:213–216
Driver (1871) Discussion: Methoden der Blepharoplastik (Knapp). Klin Monatsbl Augenheilkd 9:424
Ely ET (1881) A successful case of transplantation of skin according to Wolfe's method. Med Rec (1866–1922), 19:291
Everbusch O (1887a) Ueber die Verwendung von Epidermistransplantationen bei den plastischen Operationen an den Lidern und an der Conjunctiva. Muench Med Wochenschr 34:1–3, 19–22
Everbusch O (1887b) Discussion: Zur Operationen der Trichiasis (Vossius). Beilageheft Klin Monatsbl Augenheilkd 25:49
Fischer E (1880) Ueber die künstliche Blutleere bei der Transplantation von Hautstücken Dtsch Z Chir 13:193
Försterling K (1907) Mitteilung zur Technik der Thiersch'schen Transplantation. Zentralbl Chir 34:594
Franke E (1890) Trichiasis und Distichiasis. Muench Med Wochenschr 37:379
Hamilton FH (1871) Healing of ulcers by transplantation. NY Med J 14:225–232
von Hippel R (1887) Discussion: Zur Operation der Trichiasis (Vossius). Beilageheft Klin Monatsbl Augenheilkd 25:49
Hotz FC (1892) A few experiments with Thiersch's grafts in the operation for pterygium J Am M A 19:297–298
Horner F (1871) Discussion: Methoden der Blepharoplastik (Knapp). Klin Monatsbl Augenheilkd 9:423
Howe L (1880) Blepharoplastik durch Transplantation eines stiellosen Lappens. Zentralbl Prakt Augenheilkd 4:329
Hume GH (1882) Ectropion of both eyelids operated on by Wolfe's method. Lancet 2:100
Jaesche E (1881) Zur Trichiasis-Operation. Klin Monatsbl Augenheilkd 91:40
Kipp (1880) Discussion: Blepharoplastik durch Transplantation eines stiellosen Lappens (Howe). Zentralbl Prakt Augenheilkd 4:329
Knapp H (1880) Discussion: Blepharoplastik durch Transplantation eines stiellosen Lappens (Howe). Zentralbl Prakt Augenheilkd 4:329
Knapp H (1890) Skin-grafting on the eyelids. Med Rec (1866–1922), 38:468
Krause F Ueber die Transplantation grosser ungestielter Hautlappen. Verh Dtsch Ges Chir 1893, 22:46–51
Kuhnt H (1883) Beiträge zur operativen Augenheilkunde. Fisher, Jena
Laqueur (1887) Discussion: Zur Operation der Trichiasis (Vossius). Beilageheft Klin Monatsbl Augenheilkd 25:51
Lawson G (1870a) Cases of skin-grafting. Lancet 2:567
Lawson G (1870b) On the successful transplantation of portions of skin for the closure of large granulating surfaces. Med Times Gaz 2:631
Lawson G (1871) On the transplantation of portions of skin for closure of large granulating surfaces. Trans Clin Soc London 4:49
Lawson G (1874) Diseases and injuries of the eye. Renshaw, London
Lawson G (1882) Ectropion of the upper lid remedied by transplantating a piece of skin from the arm. Lancet 1:13–14
Le Fort L (1872) L'hétéroplastie. Bull Acad Med (Paris) 1:295
Lucas Championnière J (1888) Discussion: Greffes cutanées (Berger) Bull Soc Chir Paris 14:51
Martin G (1873) De la greffe dans le traitement de l'ectropion. Ann Oculist (Paris) 69:110
Masselon J (1875) Greffes dermiques et conjunctivales Ann Oculist (Paris) 73:131
Mathewson A (1880) Discussion: Blepharoplastik durch Transplantation eines stiellosen Lappens (Howe). Zentralbl Prakt Augenheilkd 4:329
McDowell F (1977) The source book of plastic surgery Williams & Wilkins, Baltimore

McHardy MM (1882) Successful "transportation" of skin from inner side of arm to replace skin removed with an epithelioma involving innermost third of left lower eyelid; eleven months since operation. Trans Ophthalmol Soc UK 2:5
Menzel A (1872) Kleine Beiträge zur Hauttransplantation. Wien Med Wochenschr 22:904–907
Meyer (1881) Epithéliome de l'angle interne de l'oeil gauche-abliation-greffe dermique-Guérison. Bull Soc Chir Paris 7:676
Monod Ch (1881) Sur un cas d'épithélioma de l'angle interne de l'oeil gauche, traité par le Dr. Meyer, au moyen de l'ablation et l'application d'une greffe dermique. Bull Soc Chir Paris 7:647–676
Noyes HD (1880) Formation of an eyelid. Med Rec (1866–1922) 17:344–346
Pfalz (1905) Praktische Winke für die Behandlung von Verbrennungen der Augen und Augenlider. Dtsch Med Wochenschr 31:1412–1413
Pfalz (1908) Ueber Frühtransplantation bei Verbrennungen der Augenlider. Dtsch Med Wochenschr 1:823–826
Plessing E (1888) Hautverpflanzung nach C. Thiersch. Langenbecks Arch Klin Chir 37:53–78
Raehlmann E (1891) Therapeutische Erfahrungen über Lidkanten-operation, sowie über Haut und Schleimhauttransplantation am Auge. Dtsch Med Wochenschr 17:4–9
Samelsohn (1881) Blepharoplastik mittels freier stielloser Lappenbildung. Dtsch Med Wochenschr 7:118
Schede M (1881) Die Reverdin'schen Transplantation. Dtsch Med Wochenschr 7:352
Sichel A (1875) Présentation de malades. Bull Soc Chir Paris 1:586
Silex P (1896) Ueber lidbildung mit stiellosen Hautlappen. Klin Monatsbl Augenheilkd 34:46–58
Snell S (1882) Case of ectropion successfully treated by transportation of a large non-pedicled flap from the arm. Lancet 2:102
Streatfield JF (1884) Two cases of extreme extropion of the lower lids; different operations. Trans Opthal Soc UK 4:15
Strube (1871) Discussion: Methoden der Blepharoplastik (Knapp). Klin Monatsbl Augenheilkd 9:423
Taylor CB (1875) On the transplantation of skin *en masse.* Med Times Gaz 1:18
Thiersch C (1886) Ueber Hautverpflanzung. Verh Dtsch Ges Chir 15:17–19
Toswill LH (1882) On a case of ectropion successfully treated by transplantation of skin from the arm. Br Med J 1:9–10
Urban G (1892) Ueber die Hautverpflanzung nach Thiersch. Dtsch Z Chir 34:187
Vogel K (1907) Zur Technik der Thiersch'schen Transplantation. Zentralbl Chir 34:355–357
Vossius A (1887) Zur Operation der Trichiasis; Bericht über die neunzehnte Versammlung der Ophthalmologische Gesellschaft, Heidelberg. Beilageheft Klin Monatsbl Augenheilkd 25:42
Wadsworth OF (1876) A case of ectropion treated by transplantation of a large flap without pedicle. Boston Med Surg J 95:747
de Wecker L (1872) De la greffe dermique en chirurgie oculaire. Ann Occulist (Paris) 67:62
de Wecker L (1873) Dermic grafting in ophthalmic surgery. Ophthal Hosp Rep 7:663–664
Wicherkiewicz B (1882) Zur Beurteilung des Werthes stielloser Hauttransplantationen für die Blepharoplastik. Klin Monatsbl Augenheilkd 20:419–448
Wicherkiewicz B (1887) Discussion: Zur Operation der Trichiasis (Vossius). Beilageheft Klin Monatsbl Augenheilkd 25:49
Wolfe JR (1875) A new method of performing plastic operations. Br Med J 2:360–361
Wolfe JR (1880) Ueber Lidbildung nach Wolfe's Methode. Zentralbl Prakt Augenheilkd 4:11–13
Wolfe JR (1881) On a new method of performing plastic operations. Br Med J 1:426
Wolfe JR (1882) On the transplantation of skin-flaps. Lancet 1:86
Zoltan J (1962) Die Anwendung des Spalthautlappens in der Chirurgie. Fischer, Jena
Zehender W (1879) Ueber Ektropion-Operation durch Transplantation großer Hautstücke. Klin Monatsbl Augenheilkd 22:213–222

Chapter 4
Application of the Principles of Thiersch in Skin Grafting, and Further Developments (1886–1900)

A. Skin Grafting According to the Principles of Carl Thiersch

In a previous chapter we described how skin grafts were applied to granulating wound surfaces after Reverdin's discovery (1869). After a brief period of intensive application, the interest taken in skin grafting waned markedly by about 1874. Hardly any further publications appeared in the medical journals. In fact Coombs (1876) went so far as to state: "The results of grafting pieces of living skin on wounds are so seldom made public now that the operation seems to be going out of repute."

We have also seen that one of the principal causes of the waning interest in skin grafting lay in the disappointing results as to the quality of the cicatrices. However, the interest in skin grafting revived after Thiersch delivered an address to the *Deutsche Gesellschaft für Chirurgie* [1] in 1886 (Thiersch 1886).

On that occasion, Thiersch proposed a number of essential changes in grafting.

Carl Thiersch (Fig. 16) was born in Munich, where he studied medicine. In 1843 he continued his medical training in Berlin, where he worked under Dieffenbach (1792–1847), among others. Dieffenbach let him perform several operations, and gave him an excellent testimonial when he left Berlin. Via Vienna, Thiersch went to Paris and remained there until 1847. He then returned to Munich, where he was appointed Prosector of the Institute of Pathology.

He now spent most of his time with the microscope and gave lectures on microscopic anatomy, histology and the practical use of the instrument. In those years he developed into an anatomist and in Germany as well as abroad he gradually acquired a reputation for his knowledge and skill in the field of histology; his injection specimens particularly acquired fame (von Bardeleben 1895; Garten cited by Thiersch 1922). In these, capillaries were made visible by a procedure which Thiersch himself had worked out. Thiersch did this type of investigation because of his interest in comparative anatomy. The tissues were first rendered ischaemic and then injected with coloured glue; this was followed by fixation in alcohol. The microscopic sections were cut manually by Thiersch himself (there was as yet hardly anything like a microtome). His skill in cutting sections by

1 German Surgical Society

hand must later have been very useful to Thiersch in cutting skin grafts. Jungengel (1891) later pointed out that the manual cutting of microscopic sections was the best exercise for mastering the technique of cutting free skin grafts.

In 1854, Thiersch decided henceforth to devote himself to surgery and accepted an appointment as professor of surgery in Erlangen. There he continued his studies of wound healing, publishing papers on such subjects as skin tumours and wound

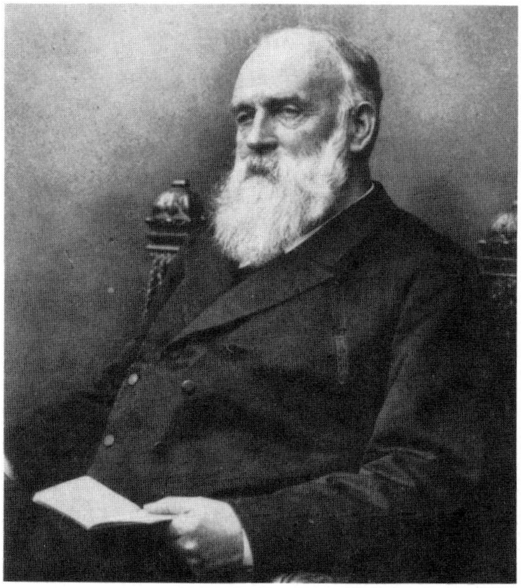

Fig. 16. Carl Thiersch (1822–1895), who played an important role in the history of skin grafting by setting up strict rules for its use

healing. In 1867 he was appointed to Leipzig. In Erlangen he was succeeded by Heineke. After Reverdin (1869) performed his first successful skin graft a few years later, Thiersch focused his attention mostly on the healing of grafts (Thierfelder 1872; Thiersch 1874).

In 1874, Thiersch had already made some cautious suggestions for improvement of results but it was not until 1886 that he reverted to this subject. This time lag is less surprising than it may seem. Thiersch was a conscientious man, who avoided hasty conclusions. Moreover, he obviously disliked publishing. His son, J. Thiersch (1922) wrote in a biography of his father that Thiersch had in fact never devoted a real publication to skin grafting. His utterances on this subject were confined to two lectures for the *Deutsche Gesellschaft für Chirurgie.*

Another fact to illustrate how selectively Thiersch used his pen, is the non-appearance of annual surveys of the surgical activities in the Leipzig Surgical Clinic, although this was customary in Germany at that time. Thiersch regarded the writing of detailed annual reports as a waste of energy rather than a contribution to science.

The lecture which Thiersch gave in 1886 comprised two subjects: rheumatoid arthritis and skin grafting. In the part on skin grafting he formulated several suggestions to improve the method, and illustrated their validity with two case histories. His recommendations boiled down to this: skin grafting should be done on a fresh wound bed; such granulation tissue as was present should be excised until a firm, freely bleeding surface was obtained.

The grafts should be split-skin grafts, always obtained from the patient himself, and should cover the entire skin defect.

In one of the two patients demonstrated by Thiersch, the upper lip had been reconstructed with the aid of a pedicled flap. The donor site and the inside of the flap had been covered with split-skin grafts. The other patient had been treated for burns: the granulation tissue had been removed, and the skin defect covered with skin grafts. After this lecture, the term "skin grafting according to Thiersch" was introduced (Sick 1887; Franke 1889). This expression has led to much misunderstanding. Thiersch only formulated certain principles of skin grafting and in his own department different views were held, certainly as regards the thickness of the grafts. In his first lecture, Thiersch himself scarcely mentioned technical details. He probably had no intention of doing so.

The Thiersch Principles Elaborated by his Pupils

It is thanks to Thiersch's pupils such as Karg (1887, 1888), Plessing (1888) and Urban (1892) that we have access to more details on the application and procedure of skin grafting as performed in Thiersch's department. Plessing described why the Reverdin method had been abandoned in Thiersch's department: firstly because the cicatrix showed severe contraction, and secondly because it was so vulnerable. Thiersch believed that in the course of wound healing, large, soft granulations were gradually converted to small, dry granulations in which few blood vessels were present. During this conversion the wound surface area diminished due to contraction of the adjacent tissues. The small, "contracting" granulations were then covered by epithelial tissue. Thiersch assumed that grafts would contract if they were applied to granulation tissue which had not yet fully contracted. If they were applied to tissue which no longer contracted, the grafts would not contract either. Thiersch held that grafting on granulation tissue had one other disadvantage: the grafts would remain vulnerable due to the softness of the underlying tissue. By removing the granulation tissue, a firm bond could be established between wound floor and graft.

Indications for Skin Grafting in Thiersch's Surgical Department

Thiersch considered fresh traumatic postoperative wounds to be very suitable for grafting. Burns were not grafted until the necrotic tissue was shed and the wound floor covered by granulation tissue. Other indications for skin grafting were ulcers of the leg and granulating defects resulting from sequestrectomy, e.g. after fractures of the lower leg.

According to Urban (1892), grafting was also done on cancellous bone, fascia, muscle tissue, tendon sheaths, perineurium, adipose tissue or cartilage. Grafting on tendon or aponeurosis was bound to fail. From 1886 to 1891, 350 grafts were performed on posttraumatic skin defects in Thiersch's surgical department. Grafting was postponed when the patient had lost too much blood. No grafts were applied to infected wounds until granulation tissue had formed. In some cases the operation had to be postponed ten to twelve weeks. Patients with burns often required reconstructive surgery, in which skin grafts were also used.

Preparation of the Wound. Thiersch made no use of antiseptic agents to cleanse the wound floor because he held that such agents as sublimate and carbolic acid (phenol) had a toxic effect. He cleansed the wound solely with saline solutions. The granulations were removed with the aid of a sharp curette, and the wound edges trimmed. The wound surface was then covered with a sponge until bleeding ceased. Haemostasis was usually achieved within 5–10 minutes. In most burn patients the operation was performed about six weeks after the accident (Plessing 1888). A few years later, operations were performed within 2–3 weeks (Urban 1892). Urban did not explain why the interval had been reduced.

Selection of the Donor Site. Thiersch had pointed out in his lecture in 1886 that all skin grafting should be done with autografts, without further explaining his remark. It was probably not fear of transmitting infections that inspired his advice. In his book *Die heteroplastische und homöoplastische Transplantation,* Schöne (1912) mentioned several times that his teacher Friedrich (who had known Thiersch as a friend) had told him how Thiersch's many experiments with homografts had all been unsuccessful. Thiersch never published any report on these experiments.

Thiersch preferred the upper arm as a donor site. In 1888, the thigh was also mentioned as a donor site (Plessing 1888). A few years later, Urban reported that for cosmetic reasons grafts were no longer taken from any site but the thigh.

Taking Grafts, Their Thickness and Dimensions. Thiersch (1886) had advised the use of one hand to flatten and stretch the skin, while the other hand cut the grafts with a razor held as flat as possible. The grafts thus obtained were 10 cm long and 2 cm wide; they consisted of epidermis, the papillary layer and part of the reticular layer. Grafts which had to be wider than 2 cm could not be taken from the upper arm lest they be too thick in the centre. The donor area was covered with iodoform, and healed within 8–10 days. Plessing maintained that this way of taking grafts was one of the major advantages of the principles outlined by Thiersch, because the donor site could be used repeatedly (three times or even more often). Partly because of this, it was not necessary to use homografts, and cross-infections were avoided. According to Plessing, the healing of the donor site occasionally took as long as 14 days.

Initially, the grafts were cut without anaesthesia (Plessing 1888). It was assumed that the patients could tolerate the procedure well. A few years later the patients were reportedly anaesthetized (Urban 1892). Thiersch still used a razor to cut grafts, but gradually more and more use was made of a long, wide, concave scalpel (Plessing 1888; Urban 1892), which was first moistened with a saline solution to facilitate cutting. The scalpel was held as flat as possible, and slow sawing movements were executed to cut a graft which, when Plessing described this in 1888, consisted of epidermis and the papillary layer (which means that at that time the grafts were cut thinner).

Even thinner grafts might possibly have been obtained by using palmar or plantar skin, but according to Thiersch this had few advantages. The cardinal point in skin grafting was to restore the vascular continuity of wound bed and graft as quickly as possible. With a graft consisting solely of epidermis, this would be much more difficult than with a thicker graft including the horizontal capillary network of the papillary layer.

Thiersch's efforts in grafting aimed at creating conditions in which the thickest possible skin graft could be expected with the greatest possible certainty to heal. The thicker the graft, the better the long-term result! It was therefore decidedly untrue that Thiersch used thin grafts, as often maintained. Undoubtedly, his pupils have also contributed to this misunderstanding. Urban stated with emphasis that the grafts had to be as thin as possible and that therefore (the technique of obtaining them being as it was in those days) the grafts could hardly be wider then 1–2 cm because, the wider the graft was cut, the thicker it had to be.

Application of the Grafts. Grafts were placed in position with the aid of a small brush or a blunt probe. The entire defect was covered with grafts. The graft edges touched each other or, sometimes, even overlapped (Plessing 1888; Urban 1892). This was to prevent the graft area from assuming a mosaic-like appearance. After application, the grafts were pressed against the underlying tissue with a spatula in order to remove blood between graft and underlying tissue and to promote adhesion.

Wet dressings were placed on the grafts to curb multiplication of bacteria. The adjacent skin was greased with oil to facilitate a change of dressing. A protective dressing of silk taffeta was applied next (Urban 1892), and this in turn was covered with a layer of cotton wool soaked in saline solution. Strips of adhesive plaster were used to fix the cotton wool. Additional compression was ensured by means of another layer of cotton wool and a circular bandage. The wet dressings were changed daily. On these occasions the wound was rinsed with a saline solution.

The use of wet dressings was discontinued after a week, because at that time healing was thought to have progressed sufficiently to prevent bacteria from exerting their influence on wound healing. The dressings were soaked loose in a bath. Infections were observed mostly in wounds which, prior to grafting, had contained pyogenic bacteria. When the wounds were not covered with dressings a layer of fibrinous tissue formed and suppuration increased markedly, causing detachment of the grafts. This experience prompted the use of dressings on all grafts.

Complications. Apart from infections in the grafted area, Plessing also described another complication, which today would probably be classified in the same category. He reported that granulation tissue sometimes grew through the grafts. This was observed in patients with osteomyelitis in whom not all sequestra had been removed. In patients with syphilitic ulcers, too, the grafts failed. Contraction occurred only if the surface had not been entirely covered with skin grafts, or if the grafting had been only partly successful.

Application of the Thiersch Principles Outside Leipzig

After Thiersch's lecture of 1886, the principles he had formulated were followed in many hospitals. At that time, the German surgeons played a prominent role. Many European and American surgeons like McBurney regularly visited Germany, and certainly attended the meetings of the *Deutsche Gesellschaft für Chirurgie.* One of the German cities where skin grafting received great attention was Erlangen. The publications of Everbusch, professor in ophthalmic surgery, Graser and Gabel, pupils of Heineke, show that transplantation enjoyed great interest. Skin grafting also received much attention in Switzerland, and particularly in Basle, in Socin's surgical department (Hübscher 1889). In France, too, the Thiersch principles were soon accepted. J. L. Reverdin's cousin Monod (1888) was especially active in this respect. Monod regarded Thiersch's advice to cover defects entirely with grafts as the principal asset of the Thiersch principles. A lecture of McBurney (1890) entitled "Experience with skin-grafting after the method of Thiersch" at a meeting of the New York Academy of Medicine revealed that the Thiersch principles had found few advocates in the United States; and this was confirmed a few years later in a lecture by Meière (1893) in which the use of the small skin grafts of Reverdin was recommended. In a patient with a skin defect resulting from contusion, 300 grafts from 10 different donors were, according to him, successfully applied within six days!

In the Netherlands, the Thiersch principles seemed to be accepted late and only with reluctance, as indicated for example in a lecture which Vermey of Amsterdam delivered in 1893 to *Het Genootschap ter bevordering der Natuur- Genees- en Heelkunde,* [2] on the subject of skin grafting (Vermey 1893). In the treatment of patients with skin defects, he used Reverdin-type autografts and homografts and also those of Thiersch. His policy was illustrated by the following case history in which only homografts were used. In an old woman with a poorly healing carbuncle, the granulation tissue was scraped off in order to apply a full-thickness homograft obtained from an amputated finger. The graft became necrotic and gradually disappeared. Next, a Thiersch skin graft was performed with an epidermal graft obtained from the foot of a three-year-old child which had been severed in a tram accident. This graft disappeared also.

Vermey did remark that the "Thiersch grafts" (he probably meant thin split-skin grafts) gave better results if obtained from the patient himself. However, he personally preferred pedicled flaps. Guldenarm (1893), who attended the lecture, disagreed. He preferred skin grafts to pedicled flaps because in his opinion the former showed no retraction and produced for that reason an equally good result.

A remarkable discussion developed after a lecture by Korteweg (1894) of Amsterdam on "The skin grafts of Thiersch". Tilanus remarked that he had always used large grafts, and had always regarded this as a well-established procedure. Korteweg remarked in reply that the Thiersch method was to be regarded as an analogue of the Reverdin method, and need not be described as a new method! In his book on general surgery, *Algemeene Heelkunde,* Korteweg (1898) described the skin grafts of

---

2 Society for the Advancement of Physics, Medicine and Surgery.

Reverdin as the method of promoting the healing of granulating wounds; he did not even mention the Thiersch principles. No uniform standpoint concerning skin grafting could be distinguished in the Netherlands at that time.

Indications for Skin Grafting. Outside Leipzig, too, indications for skin grafting did not vary widely. Grafting was done mostly in patients with posttraumatic skin defects (Knauer 1889; Ranneft 1893). Particularly in the treatment of scalp lesions sustained in machine accidents, skin grafting according to the principles of Thiersch proved to be an excellent method of ensuring rapid healing. Reimplantation of the hairy skin never led to healing (Sick 1892; Gerok 1892; Riegner 1893; Czygan 1893; Gross 1895; Altermatt 1897; Bivings 1902; Karg 1903; Mellish 1904; Enz 1905; Doering 1906; Lotheissen 1906; Miyata 1908; Robinson 1908).

Heineke (1906) removed all subcutaneous structures from the torn-off scalp and divided it into several smaller fragments. Some of these healed, but he wondered whether, in a similar future situation, he would not do better to use split-skin grafts. Grafts were applied also to skin defects resulting from tumour excision (Nagel 1889; Knauer 1889; Korteweg 1894) and in patients with ulcers resulting from specific infectious processes such as tuberculosis (Graser 1887; Jungengel 1891; Helferich 1894) or syphilis (Knauer 1889).

New indications for grafting were found in the donor sites of pedicled flaps, as Thiersch himself had also suggested (Gabel 1888; Lauenstein 1893).

Abbe (1898) used skin grafts to construct a vagina in a 21-year-old woman referred to him with vaginal agenesis (Fig. 17). Between the urethra and the anus an incision was made, and a space with a depth of 5 inches was created between bladder and rectum. A sterilized rubber cylinder filled with iodofrom gauze was covered with split-skin grafts with the under-surface turned up. Several perforations in the rubber permitted fluid to enter. This mould with skin grafts was inserted into the newly created space, to be removed after ten days. All the grafts healed. The newly created vagina was then tamponaded for four weeks. To minimize contraction the patient continued for several months to wear a mould (a wax candle was found to be most suitable for this purpose).

Skin grafts were used also to cover defects of the scalp which included the outer table of the skull (Jungengel 1891; Helferich 1894).

Thiersch grafts were regularly used in reconstructive surgery, particularly after burns. The grafts were not applied until granulation tissue had formed, at which time contractures had usually also developed.

Skin grafts were used intensively also in patients with burns. Grafting was not done until necrotic tissue was shed and granulation tissue had developed (Graser 1887; Knauer 1889; Rotgans 1893). Narath (1903) advised the use of grafts on burns on which granulation tissue had formed, not only to stop suppuration but also to improve the patient's general condition. Only when the wounds had healed did he perform "plastic operations" with the aid of single or multiple pedicled flaps to control or prevent contractures.

It was a long time before burns were treated more aggressively. Wilms (1901) [3] is usually mentioned as the first surgeon to treat burns involving full-thickness skin

---

3 The name Wilms is connected with a type of malignant kidney tumour.

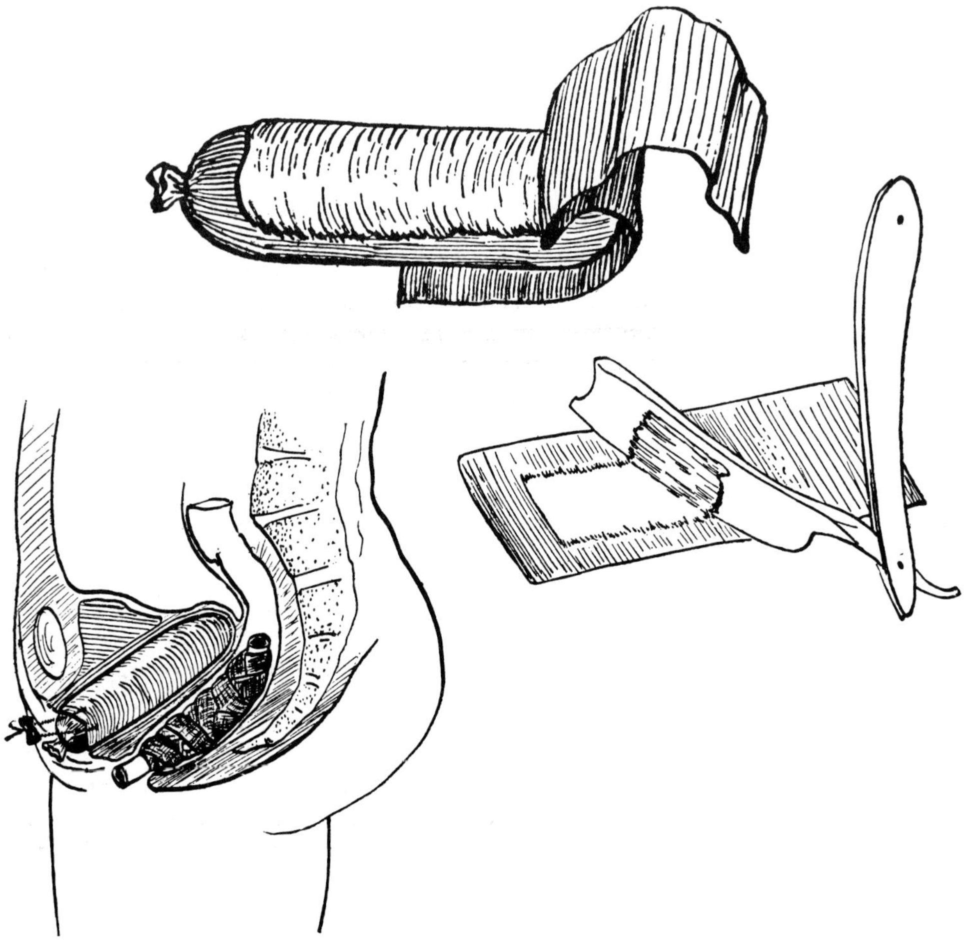

Fig. 17. Illustrations from an article of Abbe (1898) in which the use of partial-thickness skin grafts in the construction of a vagina was presented

loss by excision and immediate grafting. In an exhaustive publication on the pathology of burns Wilms devoted only a few sentences to this technique. He had noticed remarks from several sides that excision and grafting might be the only possibility of saving the lives of patients with burns. He had never heard or read that this theory had been tested in actual practice. He did treat small burns with full-thickness skin loss by excision and grafting, and the grafts healed without problems.

Hardly any mention is ever made of a report by Reahlman (1891) who, in a patient with burns of the eyelids, excised the slough on the sixth day after the accident and performed a skin graft (see Chap. 3). Since neither Raehlman's suggestion nor that of Wilms was followed, it was often necessary in burn patients to correct contractures in a second session. Several examples of this can be found.

Jüngst (1887), who saw many contractures as a result of burns of the palmar surface, used pedicled flaps from the chest to cover the skin defects resulting from excision of cicatricial tissue; and he used grafts on the donor sites. Free skin grafts were used to cover small defects of the palmar surface or the interdigital spaces. Jüngst believed that large defects could theoretically also be treated by grafting, but that the new integument was of poor quality. Heydenreich (1889) did use skin grafts to cover defects of the palmar surface. In view of the severe contractures which Jüngst had observed in patients with burns, he was inclined to attempt a more aggressive approach which, he thought, might prevent contractures. As soon as granulation tissue had formed skin grafts were applied to small defects, and pedicled flaps to large ones. Besides early operation, Heydenreich advised the use of splints, particularly in burns of the hand, to prevent contractures. Knauer (1889) stressed that grafting alone was not sufficient, and advised that active and passive exercises be started immediately after healing.

In his thesis *Ueber Prophylaxis und Therapie von Narbenkontrakturen* [4] Wauer (1893) described the use of pedicled flaps and free skin grafts in the treatment of contractures. In the case of imminent contracture, skin grafting was done as soon as possible. Nagel (1889) and Brohl (1893) used only free skin grafts in reconstruction. Brohl operated on a 3-year-old child who had developed syndactyly as a result of burns: he applied skin grafts after excising the cicatricial tissue. The result was still excellent three years after the operation.

So the results were judged more critically at that time than 20 years earlier.

Preparatory Measures. The donor site was generally cleansed with a sublimate solution (Hübscher 1889). In some cases it was first scrubbed with water and soap (König 1901). The sublimate solution was rinsed off with a sterile 0.6% NaCl solution. McBurney (1890) advised the use of a mercurous chloride solution to cleanse the donor area. After excision of the grafts, the donor site was covered with a dressing because the patients then complained less of a burning, painful sensation (Jungengel 1891).

Thiersch (1886) had advised against the use of antiseptic solutions in the preparation of wounds for grafting. He thought that these solutions had a toxic effect on the wound bed. Several surgeons disagreed with Thiersch, e.g. Knauer (1889) assistant of Schönborn, professor of surgery in Würzburg, and McBurney. Knauer cleaned the wounds with carbolized water, and McBurney used a mercurous chloride solution. Jungengel, another assistant of Schönborn investigated the question whether 2% carbolic acid (phenol) solution or 0.1% sublimate solution had a toxic effect or exerted an unfavourable influence on wound healing. In his clinical studies he used grafts immersed in these solutions, and found that healing was not unfavourably influenced.

Thiersch's advice to remove granulation tissue, was initially followed carefully (Jeaschke 1887; Monod 1888; Knauer 1889; Jalaguier 1889). Graser (1887) also removed the granulation tissue, but wondered why he did this, for he observed that new granulation tissue formed beneath the grafts and raised its surface by as much as 3–4 mm.

4 On the prevention and treatment of cicatricial contractures.

Ollier (1889) complained that he had proposed the removal of granulation tissue as early as 1871 but that Thiersch, who had not done this until 1886, was honoured for it. It is difficult to understand that Ollier also stated that Thiersch's suggestion always to remove granulation tissue, made no sense!

Gradually, more and more voices were raised against removal of granulation tissue, because the result was not unfavourably influenced by it (Jungengel 1891; Helferich 1894; Schnitzler and Ewald 1894; Köhler 1898a; Lauenstein 1904; Isnardi 1905). Isnardi (1905) probably had the most extensive experience in this respect. He had performed skin grafts on 140 patients in the course of eight years. At a follow-up long after grafting, he found a firm scar showing no tendency to contract, although granulation tissue had not been removed. The integument was movable in relation to the underlying structure. Isnardi contended that Thiersch's advice not to graft until six weeks after formation of granulation tissue had been wrong.

In the Netherlands, too, Thiersch's advice does not seem to have been much heeded (Vermey 1893; Korteweg 1894; Tilanus 1894; Loopuyt 1903; Narath 1903).

Thickness and Dimensions of the Grafts. Skin grafting was done more and more under general anaesthesia (Everbusch 1887; Graser 1887; Gabel 1888; McBurney 1890). Jungengel (1891) reported that grafting was initially done under general anaesthesia, but subsequently without anaesthesia because anaesthesia was considered superfluous: the patients had no pain when the grafts were excised-merely a sensation of being shaved not too expertly. The advantage of operating on a conscious patient was that he contracted his muscles, which facilitated excision of the graft.

Hübscher (1889) was among the first to report explicitly that his operations were performed under aseptic precautions (in 1887, von Bergmann had introduced sterilization with the aid of steam). The Thiersch principles were more or less followed. Virtually all surgeons preferred autografts. In France, such authors as Lucas Championnière[5] (1888) and Ollier (1889) pointed out that homografts were useless. The former reported that homografts initially seemed to heal like autografts, but disappeared completely after 6–8 weeks. Ollier maintained that homografts disappeared as a result of absorption. McBurney always used autografts himself, but thought that homografts might be used just as well.

Although there was a consensus of opinion about the use of autografts, other aspects of skin grafting were more controversial, e.g. the question of the proper graft thickness. Everbusch, Graser and Gabel intimated that they used thinner grafts than Thiersch, initially not on principle but for practical reasons: they did not have the instruments required to cut grafts of fair thickness. They used the knife which Katsch had designed for the microtome. The grafts they obtained with this knife were so thin as to be transparent. The donor site showed little bleeding. Microscopic examination revealed that the grafts consisted of epidermis and the top surface of the papillary layer.

5 Lucas Championnière was one of the first French surgeons who applied antisepsis in surgical management.

The cutting of these grafts was difficult and time-consuming. The grafts measured 3×1 cm. Everbusch reached the conclusion that these grafts had many advantages. He maintained that the Malpighian layer was the principal component of the graft; the closer the Malpighian layer and the underlying structure were together, the more effective the plasma circulation should be and the more reliable the adhesion of the graft to the underlying structure. The grafts used by Hübscher and Jungengel likewise consisted only of epidermis and papillary layer. They preferred these grafts for the same reason as Everbusch (see Fig. 18). In Germany, the thin grafts were known as *Thiersch grafts.* Both Jaeschke

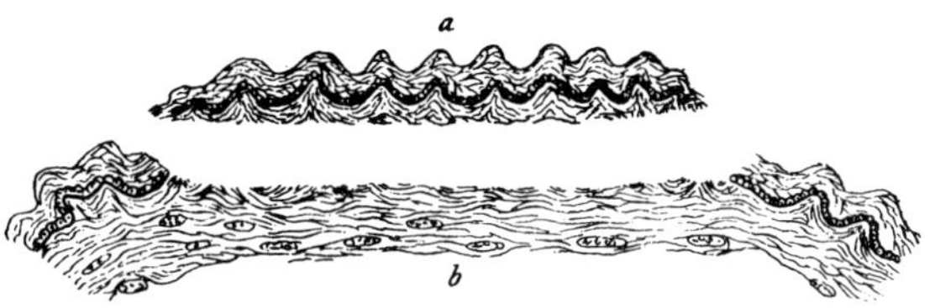

Fig. 18. The thickness of skin grafts as were cut by Hübscher (1889). The grafts consisted of epidermis and a thin layer of corium

and Knauer believed that Thiersch cut his grafts as thin as possible. Hübscher and Jungengel both stressed that Thiersch used grafts consisting of epidermis, papillary layer and part of the reticular layer, whereas they themselves used thinner grafts. Jungengel cut grafts no wider than 1 cm with a specially designed scalpel (when the grafts were wider they were also thicker, and contained the reticular layer). But a change of technique made it possible to cut wider thin grafts. This was achieved mainly by having an assistant stretch the skin and flatten the area of operation (Hübscher 1889; Fig. 19).

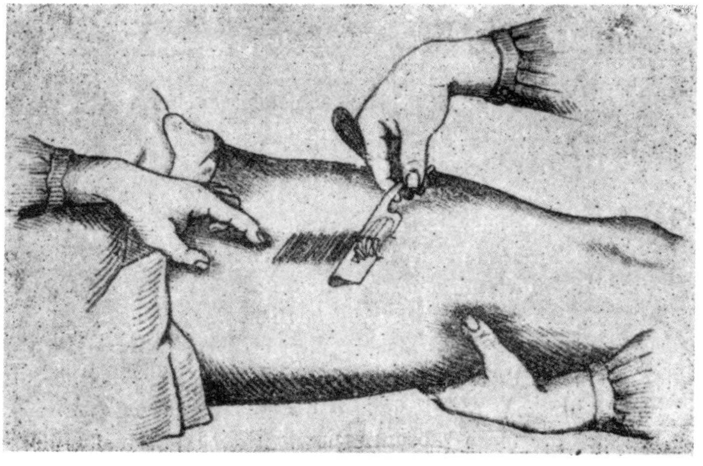

Fig. 19. The hand of an assistant stretched the skin of the donor area to facilitate the cutting of the grafts (Hübscher 1889)

Hübscher used both the microtome knife and a razor to cut grafts. Monod also preferred the microtome knife. This was not surprising because Monod had learnt the technique from Socin in Basle, where Hübscher also worked. Monod, too, obtained thinner grafts with the microtome knife than Thiersch had used. It is unlikely that the grafts which Thiersch cut were quite as thick as Pozzi (1888) described. Pozzi had visited Thiersch's department and claimed to have adopted his principles. When he had cut his grafts, he could close the donor site with sutures! Heydenreich (1889), who had also visited Thiersch, likewise found the grafts too thick. He preferred the grafts cut in Socin's department in Basle.

The grafts which Ollier preferred and which he called "greffes autoplastiques", probably consisted of epidermis and the entire corium. These grafts were probably of the same thickness as those he described in 1872: fairly thick at the centre, and thin at the periphery.

Special mention should be made of Obst (1894), who worked in von Bardeleben's department in Berlin. He wrote a thesis entitled *Beitrag zur Transplantation dicker Hautlappen* [6]. He considered that the thin skin grafts of Everbusch, or even the thicker grafts used by Thiersch, produced disappointing results. The grafted area remained vulnerable after healing, and the cosmetic result was poor. On the other hand, full-thickness grafts also had their disadvantages. Immediately after excision their dimensions often diminished considerably, so that the skin defects caused were much larger than the area to be grafted. The donor site had to be closed with sutures, and the technique of full-thickness skin grafting was difficult. Obst therefore devised the use of "thick" grafts which resembled full-thickness grafts as to results, but split-skin grafts as to the technique of excision and application. He used a razor to cut grafts with a length of 4–5 cm and a width of 2–3 cm, which comprised nearly the entire thickness of the skin. The donor site was then painted with 1% silver nitrate and powdered with bismuth subnitrate. The dressing remained in situ for two to three weeks, after which the donor site had by no means always healed. The results obtained with these grafts were very good.

Application of the Grafts. One of the principal criteria applied to the wound bed was that it should be dry. Bleeding beneath a graft was regarded as a serious complication, because the accumulation of blood prevented rapid attachment. Everbusch (1887) attached so much importance to a dry wound bed that he sometimes waited 6–7 hours before grafting. During this interval the grafts were often kept in a 0.6% NaCl solution. Trnka (1893) and Obst (1894) also waited a few hours (5–6) in some cases. Obst rarely applied the skin grafts immediately after removal of the granulation tissue. He sometimes used bellows to dry the wound surface!

The grafts were applied to the wound floor with the aid of all sorts of simple instruments such as dissecting needles (Hübscher 1889; Fig. 20), cataract needles (Monod 1888) or a probe and tweezers (König 1901).

Nearly all surgeons covered the entire wound bed with grafts, as Thiersch had advised. Everbusch in addition ensured that the skin pattern of the graft corresponded with that of the skin to be replaced.

---

6 Contribution to the use of thick skin grafts.

Wound Dressing After Grafting. Although nearly all surgeons applied some kind of dressing after grafting, the question gradually arose whether "open" wound management would be possible. Reverdin (1876), Hübscher (1889) and Jungengel (1891) had already suggested that this might be quite possible.

Brüning (1904) is generally given the merit of having been the first to use "open wound management" systematically. He had adopted this idea from Wagner (1903) and Bernhard (1904), who left granulating wounds without dressing. Brüning did

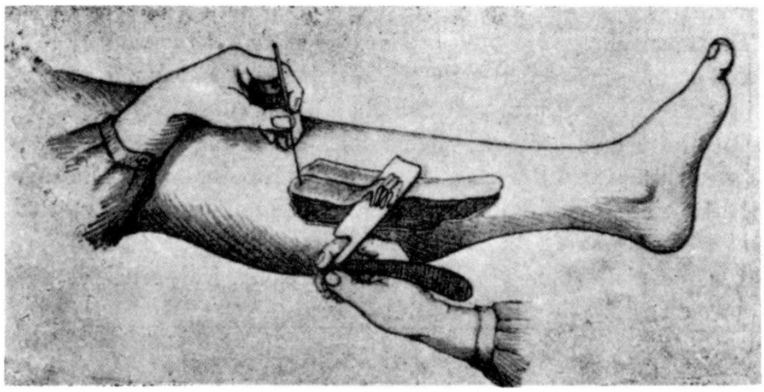

Fig. 20. Several simple instruments were used to position the skin grafts; in this case dissecting needles (Hübscher 1889)

the same in cases in which grafting had been done under local anaesthesia. In some cases the patients were left on the table for hours after the operation, to ensure adequate adhesion of the graft to the underlying structure. The uncovered wounds sometimes produced serous fluid; when this accumulated beneath the grafts, it was drained off. The wounds were dressed at night to prevent displacement of the grafts due to unexpected movements of the sleeping patient. The advantage of open management was believed to lie in prevention of damage and displacement caused by the dressing. The risks involved in frequent changes of dressing were accepted.

Weischer (1906) obtained disappointing results with open management. Goldmann (1906) replied to Weischer's publication and wrote that open management was of importance especially during the first few hours after grafting. During that time the layer between graft and wound floor had a chance to dry, ensuring good adhesion of the grafts to the underlying structures. Once this had been established, he believed, the grafted areas could well be dressed.

Several techniques of wound dressing were used. In Everbusch's ophthalmological department in Erlangen, the grafts were initially powdered with chloroform and then covered with wet dressings. The wound was inspected after 8–10 days, whereupon open management followed. Another method used in the same department was to cover the grafts with gutta-percha, with a compression bandage on top. This led to disappointing results because the grafts were displaced beneath the bandage (Gabel 1888).

Aids other than gutta-percha were also used to prevent adhesion of the graft to the dressing. An example was tin foil (Monod 1888; Jungengel 1891), which was then covered with gauze, sometimes soaked in sublimate solution (Jungengel 1891) or saline solution (Obst 1894), or with dry iodoform gauze (Monod 1888). Gradually, dressings which ensured adequate drainage were introduced, e.g. perforated silk taffeta (Jaeschke 1887; Knauer 1889).

Kuhn (1906) and Waljaschko (1906) used tulle for dressing; when the grafts were below the level of the skin, enough tulle was applied to neutralize the difference. The dressing was left in situ for 8–10 days. Waljaschko used collodion to fix the tulle around the graft. McBurney (1890), who used a tourniquet for grafting, left the cuff in position while he applied the dressing and one or two hours afterwards, to ensure optimal adhesion between graft and wound bed.

Postoperative Treatment and Results of Skin Grafting. After the introduction of the Thiersch principles, no more was published about postoperative management than after Reverdin's invention. Jaeschke of Hamburg recommended in 1887 that, after healing, the grafted area be massaged to improve the quality of the scar as long as the patient was confined to bed (he did not specify the duration of this period). He did state that the development of a dark-blue colour under the grafted area should be considered a dangerous symptom when the patient was mobilized. The vitality of the graft was threatened in such cases.

The desquamation which sometimes occurred with inconvenient intensity after grafting, was treated by Jaeschke by scrubbing with water and soap, whereupon the grafts were greased with lanolin or petroleum jelly. Jungengel likewise observed this intensive desquamation after grafting, but believed that it ceased spontaneously (it sometimes also disappeared after application of olive oil). He, too, thought that massage had a favourable effect on desquamation. Goldmann (1894) working in the surgical clinic of Professor Kraske in Freiburg, examined the scales, which proved to consist of a keratin-like substance. He found that desquamation ceased spontaneously a few months after grafting, but reported greasing with castor oil had a favourable effect. In his opinion the desquamation resulted from a change in the nutrition of the epidermis.

Another widely discussed consequence of grafting was the highly controversial question whether the grafts did or did not contract. Jungengel, who described the results obtained in 93 patients with failures in 5%, concluded that contraction of the grafts ultimately occurred in nearly all cases. He assumed that the degree of contraction was related to the thickness of the granulation tissue (if it had not been removed) and the flexibility and mobility of the adjacent skin. If the adjacent skin had been fixed to the underlying tissues, contraction could even remain entirely absent. He also concluded that, in the patients he had treated, grafting on fresh wounds had caused more contraction than grafting on granulating surfaces. Perhaps, he thought, this was because the contraction had already occurred in the granulating wounds. Several surgeons, e.g. Helferich of Greifswald in 1894 and Isnardi working in the S. Giovanni Hospital in Turin in 1905 disagreed with him on this point. They observed no contraction after grafting on fresh wounds, nor after grafting without removal of granulation tissue.

Ollier (1898 a, b) thought differently about the contraction of grafts. In fact he maintained that a graft could increase in size.

A 55-year-old man had sustained burns of the leg at the age of 5. The burns had never healed completely, and a carcinoma had developed in the defect. Excision of this tumour caused a skin defect of 200 cm^2. One half of the defect was immediately covered with grafts, and the other half four weeks later. Ollier used skin of varying thickness in these operations. Some parts of the graft comprised only part of the thickness of the skin, and other parts comprised the full thickness. The part of the wound to which grafts were applied after four weeks contained granulation tissue. The grafts all healed. Four and a half years later the grafted area was hardly distinguishable from adjacent regions. The cicatrix was flexible and movable, and showed a normal colour. Normal hairs grew on it. Sensibility was likewise normal. Ollier had noticed that the grafted area had increased in size during these four and a half years. He could not explain this, but assumed that increased nutrition or interstitial hyperplasia of the grafted tissues could have played a role.

Since the patient described by Ollier showed hair growth in the grafted area, we may assume that he had mainly used full-thickness skin grafts.

Isnardi (1905), who used thinner grafts, observed that only protective sensibility was restored.

Reports on long-term results of grafting were generally scanty. Even in the thesis of König (1901) with the promising title *Zur Kenntnis der Dauer Resultate nach Hauttransplantation* [7], the period of observation proved always to have been less than one year. One of the few to study long-term results was Goldmann (1894). He was interested in healing long after grafting, and was surprised that the grafts became so flexible 6–8 weeks after application. In some cases the grafted skin could even be moved over the underlying structures. The size of the skin defect and the quality of the adjacent tissues played a role in this respect.

Goldmann assumed that, when transplanted skin could be moved in relation to the underlying tissues, elastic fibres had to be present; he believed that regeneration of elastic fibres started immediately after grafting and that the fibres entered the graft from the tissue beneath the graft or from the wound edges. Regeneration, he thought, did not cease until after several weeks and could be inhibited by granulation tissue. Since in his opinion the quality of the cicatrix largely depended on the amount of elastic fibres, all factors had to be eliminated which might prevent the entry of elastic fibres, e.g. infections and bleeding. The elastic fibres could prevent contraction.

Goldmann also studied the recovery of sensory perception in grafts. In grafts which had healed uneventfully, it took two or three months before tactile, thermal or pain stimuli could be perceived. Sensibility was first restored at the periphery of the graft. At the centre, islands of sensibility later appeared which increased in size and gradually merged. Regeneration of nerve terminals was believed to take place from the wound floor and the adjacent tissues. The graft healing process lasted many weeks to months. During this period the graft was still vulnerable and had to be handled with care.

Results of Skin Grafting in Ulcers of the Leg. At the time of Reverdin, skin grafting was regarded as the treatment of choice for ulcers of the leg, even though it led to many disappointments. When Thiersch (1886) presented his new principles it was believed by many that a better therapeutic method had been found. This is

7 On long-term results of skin grafting.

illustrated in an enthusiastic publication by Jaeschke (1887); he regarded skin grafting as the treatment of choice for ulcers of the leg because he believed that ulcers would heal within a short time and that no relapses would occur. Less positive publications soon followed.

Nagel (1889) reported that the ulcers relapsed after some time, which did not surprise him very much because the local vascularization and the callous aspect of the ulcers held little promise of a lasting cure. It did surprise Nagel that he was the only one to have obtained disappointing results. He suspected that others had reported only short-term results, and this suspicion was confirmed in a postscript to a publication by Franke (1889). He, too, initially seemed to have obtained good results, but he observed relapses after 3–9 months. Jungengel (1891) reported ulcer relapses after six months in his patients. In about 50% of his patients, Garrè (1889) observed the same complication after a few weeks to months.

Histological examination showed that two processes were the cause. In some of his failures, Garrè observed leucocyte infiltrates beneath the grafts and he assumed that this was due to some kind of inflammation. In other patients he found accumulation of blood or blood pigment beneath the grafts. The blood vessels showed total or partial damage, and the distal ends of the capillaries were dilatated and blood-filled. Garrè thought that the ultimate destruction of the graft resulted from insufficient blood supply. Helferich (1894) tried to prevent relapses by prescribing prolonged bed rest; he applied a zinc gelatin dressing before he allowed his patients up. Köhler (1898 a), a former assistant of von Bardeleben, considered venous insufficiency to be the cause of relapse of ulcers. In patients with venous ulcers he therefore first excised a small segment of the great saphenous vein and removed varicose veins before he excised the ulcer. Several of the ulcers thus treated healed. If they did not, a skin graft was applied to the granulation tissue. The patients were confined to bed during treatment. The results were nevertheless disappointing, because the patients wanted to go home and did so as soon as they saw that the grafts had healed. They usually started walking prematurely, and the grafts were often damaged as a result. Blood-filled blisters formed in the grafted area. Köhler ascribed this to insufficient fibrosis of the granulation tissue. By intervening immediately and prescribing a strict regimen of bed rest, elevation of the leg and compression bandages, he was usually able to save those parts of the graft that had remained intact.

Another publication by Köhler (1898 b) shows that skin grafts were subsequently used in only a few patients with ulcers of the leg. Karewski (1898) replied to Köhler's publication: he believed that grafts could quite well be applied to granulation tissue, but that in that case the relapse rate was higher than that in patients in whom the granulation tissue had been excised.

In the Netherlands, too, the results of skin grafting in ulcers of the leg were disappointing (Korteweg 1893). Vermey (1893) believed that there was no correlation between ulcer relapse and grafts. In this context he quoted Koch, Professor of Surgery in Groningen, who had successfully treated an extensive ulcer by skin grafting (a new ulcer had subsequently formed, but the grafted area had remained intact).

The full-thickness skin graft had meanwhile also been used widely in the treatment of ulcers of the leg, and had likewise failed to give satisfactory results

(Karg 1888; Henle and Wagner 1899). Wagner, assistant of Mikulicz in Breslau, reported that full-thickness skin grafting had failed in two-thirds of his patients with ulcers of the leg. In four of his 22 patients, a relapse had subsequently occurred (Henle and Wagner 1899). He agreed with Karg (1888) that skin grafting in ulcers of the leg was merely a symptomatic treatment.

Healing After Split-Skin Grafting

Wound healing was intensively studied by Garrè (1889), Jungengel (1891), Enderlen (1897) of Marburg and Marchand (1901) of Leipzig. The Swiss Garrè, who worked in Tübingen (Germany) under Bruns and had previously worked in Socin's hospital in Basle (Switzerland), was one of the first to publish a systematic study. Although his publication was entitled *Ueber die histologischen Vorgänge bei der Anheilung der Thiersch'schen Transplantationen* [8], he stated in the introduction that the grafts studied had been thinner than those used by Thiersch. The study comprised a series of 35 cases in which graft healing had been studied from five and a half hours to two and a half years after the operation.

Changes in the Wound Bed. Fairly soon after grafting, a layer of erythrocytes became visible between graft and wound bed. The erythrocytes were embedded in a network of fibrin. The thickness of the layer varied markedly, but it was usually twice as thick as the graft (Jungengel 1891). Within 24 hours, this layer contained more leucocytes than erythrocytes. Leucocyte infiltration was most pronounced after two or three days. The leucocytes contained nuclear particles or remnants of pigment. The erythrocytes disintegrated and the fibrin began to dissolve. During the first 48 hours, many leucocytes were observed around the capillaries of the wound surface also (Jungengel 1891; Enderlen 1897). Garrè observed fibroblast formation within 24 hours of grafting; he assumed that the fibroblasts produced granulation tissue. Jungengel postulated that leucocytes, giant cells or capillaries had to do with the formation of granulation tissue. The giant cells disappeared again when the granulation tissue was converted to connective tissue. The layer of exudate gradually assumed the character of a germinal layer, and after two to four days showed proliferation of thin-walled sprig-like blood vessels which linked the vessels of the wound bed to those of the graft. In the case of a thick graft, the leucocytes in the exudate or germinal layer persisted much longer than in that of a thin graft. An exudate layer did not even form when epithelium was in direct contact with the wound bed. According to Garrè, the exudate layer disappeared in about 14 days; according to Jungengel this took only six days.

Changes in the Graft. Some of the blood vessels of the graft became involved in the circulation after two or three days (Garrè 1889; Jungengel 1891). Prior to that time, no blood entered the newly fromed capillaries. Garrè as well as Jungengel assumed that the graft survived that period via "endo-osmotic" fluid exchange, even though Garrè did not exclude the possibility that leucocytes might also play a role in nutrition. Karg (1887, 1888) and Jungengel maintained that the pigmented

---

8 "Histological processes in the healing of Thiersch grafts."

cells in the epithelial layer of the graft might also play a role in nutrition. The first signs of degeneration of epidermis occurred after three or four days.

According to Garrè, the top layer of the Malpighian layer detached itself. Marchand suspected that Garrè had made a mistake and really meant the epidermis. Jungengel wrote that the horny layer became detached on the fourth day, so that intercellular bridges became visible. Vesicular changes developed in the epithelium (Jungengel 1891; Marchand 1901). According to Jungengel, these vesicular changes used to be interpreted as indicating insufficient nutrition if seen in other conditions. The middle layers of the epidermis also changed. The cell nuclei shrank and responded more intensively to histological staining. The cells of the Malpighian layer resumed their mitotic activity once circulation was restored (Garrè 1889).

The cells of this layer were narrow and cylindrical so that the bottom layers were arranged perpendicular to the surface. The nuclei were small and stained dark. Mitotic activity was maximal at sites where the Malpighian layer had been severed and at the sites of hair follicles and sweat glands. From the wound edges, too, bulbous proliferations with epithelium entered. The floor was thus filled up with epithelial cells, which ensured a firm link between the layer with exudate and the graft.

Once the epithelial cells reached the layer with fibrin, they accumulated along the irregular surface and pushed the fibrin layer away; or they slipped between the fibrin layer and the wound bed. From the second postoperative day on, leucocytes also became visible in the epidermis. According to Marchand, the nearly circular defects in the epidermis resulted from degeneration and serous imbibition. Leucocytes accumulated in these defects, and round cells were present in the crevices between dermis and epidermis. The dermis already showed degenerative changes during the first days after grafting, and these were accompanied by increasing infiltration of polynuclear round cells (leucocytes) which extended as far as the papillae and the epithelium. There seemed to be a correlation between the number of leucocytes and the degree of epithelial degeneration and necrosis. The number of leucocytes diminished when epithelial necrosis was complete. The nuclei of the connective tissue cells already showed partial shrinking on the second day. They stained dark and presented a lobular appearance.

Part of these cells remained intact. In the deeper dermal layers, more and more apparently young fusiform cells were formed. It was difficult to establish whether they had formed at this site or had entered from the underlying structures. The connective tissue fibres were more or less swollen or seemed disintegrated. Leucocytes were often also seen in tissue interstices. The young tissue subsequently increased in volume, and mitotic activity intensified. During the first few days, the blood vessels in the dermis showed evidence of degeneration. In the vessels which remained intact, vital red blood corpuscles which must have come from elsewhere became visible. In a very early phase – within two days according to Enderlen (1897) – the blood vessels could be filled with contrast medium. (Blue gum was used for this purpose. This substance was injected by Marchand, Chief of the Institute of Pathology. In 1900 Marchand was appointed to Leipzig.) These vessels communicated with the underlying structures. How this communication was established, however, remained obscure.

Marchand pointed out that vascular buds on two apposed wound surfaces also established communication, and he supposed that something similar happened after skin grafting. Abundant vascular buds developed from the underlying structures within the first few days. When the blood vessels in the superficial and middle layers of the skin graft had become necrotic, erythrocytes could nevertheless enter them because part of their endothelium had remained intact. A new endothelial tube could be formed from the intact endothelium within a short time. In that case it was difficult to establish whether an old or a newly formed blood vessel was seen in a section. On the other hand, vascular buds from the underlying structures could grow directly into the graft vessels so that a new vessel formed in a degenerated endothelial tube.

The blood vessels in the graft were initially wide, but subsequently seemed to diminish in width. The changes were related to the graft thickness, the quality of the wound bed, and the thickness of the fibrin layer. The changes in the collagen fibres and in the elastic fibers did not take a parallel course. According to Enderlen, the elastic fibres remained intact longer. Five days after grafting they were pushed apart and their arrangement became more and more irregular. The elastic fibres had virtually disappeared after 21 days. Only small lumps of degenerated fibres were present at scattered sites, and an occasional intact fibre was visible. The symptoms of degeneration were demonstrated by the feeble histological staining and fragmentation of the fibres.

Degeneration usually started in the smaller fibres. The elastic fibres were pushed away by granulation tissue, and formation of new elastic fibres did not start until after about 30 days. Elastic fibres were again present in abundance three months after the operation, but they were less regularly arranged than those in normal skin. According to Enderlen, the new fibres originated from the adjacent tissues; in his opinion old fibres could not (or perhaps could only rarely) be a point of departure or regeneration. Marchand opposed this view; in his opinion the elastic fibres in the graft were completely remodelled.

The behaviour of the collagen fibres was quite different from that of the elastic fibres. The collagen fibres regenerated within nine days of the operation.

Goldmann (1894) studied wound healing three to five months after grafting and found that regeneration of blood vessels was still in progress at that time. Immediately beneath the basal layer, these vertical blood vessels ramified in a horizontal plane and formed anastomoses with adjacent vessels. The vessels had adapted themselves to the size of the papillae. After three to five months the transition from wound bed to graft still showed cavities of an irregular shape and lined with a thin layer of epithelium, sometimes even with adventitia. Goldmann assumed that these cavities were old, dilated lymph vessels rather than old degenerated blood vessels, as others suggested. The 6 months which Goldmann spend with Weigert, one of the founders of the histological colour techniques, proved to be useful in his studies on healing of skin grafts.

Nearly all investigators concluded from their findings that thin grafts were preferable to thick grafts. The former were more easily applied to an irregular wound bed, so that a thinner fibrin layer formed. The circulation in thin grafts was more readily restored, and healing was therefore quicker. The quality of the ultimate integument was not considered in these statements.

Preservation of Skin Grafts

Surgeons concerning themselves with skin grafting soon raised the question of how long the skin remained vital after interruption of the circulation. This was initially an important question because during the period 1869–1886 use was made chiefly of homografts obtained from amputated limbs or from cadavers.

One of the first to study the vitality of skin grafts systematically was the American surgeon Brewer of Norwich, Connecticut in 1882. He obtained skin from cadavers or amputated limbs, but unfortunately he did not specify the size and thickness of the grafts he used. The skin graft was wrapped in paper or gauze and then stored – sometimes in the surgeon's pocket (!) and sometimes in a cupboard or in some special, cool place. The interval between obtaining the graft and applying it ranged from 18 to 45 hours. In one case a graft had been obtained 17 hours after the donor's death, homografting being done 24 hours later. On the basis of his experiments, Brewer concluded that (homo)grafting could be done up to 36 hours after amputation or the donor's death. Grafts with skin obtained later, failed. Brewer maintained that this was due to insufficient vitality of the grafts (Brewer 1882).

The criteria of "vitality" of skin were not defined in Brewer's publication; the ability of the graft to heal was probably the sole criterion. Ignoring the publication by Brewer, Wentscher (1894) of Thorn (Germany) is usually mentioned as the first investigator to study the duration of the suitability of a skin fragment for grafting. The purpose of Wentscher's study was to establish whether skin could be stored without disadvantages "until the wound was ready for grafting". Everbusch (1887) had previously reported that he stored grafts for 6–7 hours before applying them. He postponed grafting until he was sure that the wound was no longer bleeding. Like Everbusch, Wentscher kept the grafts in a 0.6% NaCl solution. During the winter, the graft in the NaCl solution was placed near a stove to keep it warm.

In Wentscher's first experiments, the grafts were usually stored for 24 hours (the longest period was 50 hours). Before applying them, they were washed with a 0.5–1% Lysol solution! Wentscher was satisfied with the results in 16 patients. He concluded that skin preserved for 24–48 hours was as suitable for grafting as fresh skin, but he did not specify his criteria in the evaluation of the results. A modern reader will find it strange that Wentscher also described favourable results after homografting even after grafting on compact bone without periosteum.

Wentscher (1898) subsequently studied the question of whether grafts could be preserved dry. He kept some of his grafts in a saline solution, and wrapped others in dry sterile gauze. The latter grafts were "soaked" in a saline solution before application. Most grafts were applied to the wound after 24 hours, but some were preserved for a much longer period. Wentscher even described a successful graft after preservation for 22 days (he did not mention in which manner this graft was preserved, probably in the 0.6% NaCl solution). In sections cut four days after grafting, he observed cell division in the basal layer. But this was not seen in grafts which had been preserved for 28–34 days.

Wentscher noticed that skin could easily resist cold. Storage of skin at –50 °C for 14 hours did not affect its vitality. Heat was much less well tolerated, although skin heated at 50 °C for 15 minutes was accepted. The grafts proved to be very sensitive to chemicals. Their vitality was destroyed by antiseptic agents.

Wentscher's findings were criticized. Marchand (1901) wrote that, in spite of the "careful and scientific set-up" of Wentscher's experiments, his results raised doubts and were suggestive of errors of evaluation.

Enderlen (1898), who repeated Wentscher's experiments at Marchand's request, was unable to reproduce Wentscher's results as to the survival of skin preserved dry. In no case did he observe acceptance of a dry partial-thickness skin graft. He believed that Wentscher had been misled by the colour and the adhesion of these grafts, which had simulated healing. Enderlen illustrated his point with several examples. A skin fragment applied after 24 hours' dry preservation seemed to be accepted, but examination of the grafted area excised 18 days after the operation failed to reveal even a trace of epithelial regeneration.

Enderlen agreed with Wentscher that skin preserved in saline solution remained suitable for grafting for some time. A graft preserved in saline solution for four days was accepted although most of it became necrotic and far less epithelium was formed than in a fresh graft. There was a difference in healing between fresh and preserved grafts. These differences were most evident in the corium. The corium of preserved grafts no longer contained live cells, whereas that of fresh grafts probably did. Epithelial regeneration was much slower in preserved than in fresh grafts.

Ljunggren (1898) also studied the time during which epithelial components remained vital in skin not supplied with blood. He preserved split-skin grafts in ascites fluid at room temperature, over a period ranging from two days to six months. The grafts were then examined microscopically. Symptoms of degeneration were observed in the superficial layers of epidermis. The horny layer had detached itself, sometimes together with the entire epithelial layer. The deeper layers of epidermis still contained well-preserved cells with normal nuclei after as long as three months, although the cells did show atrophy. The vitality was tested by grafting. Of the 22 grafts, 11 healed well; three of these had been preserved for four weeks. Ljunggren concluded that skin could survive preservation and retained its ability to form epithelial cells. He wondered whether better media might be found for skin preservation, and whether it might not be better to keep the grafts in an environment with a low temperature!

Marchand (1901) severely criticized Ljunggren's studies, which he described as uncertain and incomplete. Ljunggren's suggestion that it might be advisable to keep the grafts cool, had already been put into practice by Henle (1898) in the surgical clinic of Mikulicz in Breslau. He stored skin in a saline solution placed during 48 hours in a refrigerator (i.e. a cabinet chilled with ice) and then used it for grafting. Henle must therefore have been one of the first to keep grafts cool.

Burkhardt (1905a, b) likewise studied skin survival, but he preserved his specimens differently. He used canine instead of human skin, and preserved it at 12 °C in either a dry or a moist environment through which extra oxygen was passed. The dry or moist grafts retained their normal anatomy for three or four days, whereupon signs of degeneration developed; the nearly cubical epithelial cells flattened. The grafting of this canine skin on other dogs caused so many practical problems that the further findings hardly warranted any conclusions. For example, attempts to graft skin preserved for four, five or seven days failed, but skin preserved in a moist environment for eight days was successfully grafted. One graft, preserved in a dry environment for twelve days and then applied, was reportedly also accepted. According to Burkhardt, the principal sign of vitality of a graft was the ability of the epithelium to form offshoots, particularly from the deeper layers. He regarded firm, evenly distributed adhesion of graft to wound bed as another sign of vitality. It surprised Burkhardt that the method of preservation did not seem to be very important, although complete dehydration of the grafts had to be avoided. On microscopic examination he observed few differences between skin preserved dry and that preserved moist. In view of his findings he doubted Thiersch's hypothesis that during the first two or three days after grafting, skin lived on "plasmatic circulation". Although graft tissues had undoubtedly imbibed plasma, he did not accept this as proof of nutrition supplied by plasma. In his opinion it was equally possible that the cells survived by virtue of their own reserves. He maintained that the cells of the basal layer could survive the longest period without nutrition. He thought that two factors explained this: this layer contained the youngest cells, which were bound to survive relatively longer, and after prolonged preservation of the grafts these cells did not lose their original structure (whereas the other cells did). Burkhardt reached the conclusion that skin grafts preserved for one or two days survived. He probably meant that the basal layer retained its ability to form new epithelial cells. He maintained that it made no sense to preserve grafts longer than 24–36 hours. He advised that grafts should not be applied immediately to fresh wound surfaces but to wait 24 hours, because during this period a thin layer of granulation tissue was formed to which the grafts firmly adhered.

B. Grafting Epithelial Scrapings

Von Mangoldt of Dresden thought in 1895 that grafting as done by Thiersch and others had disadvantages. It required surgical skill to cut the grafts, the entire defect had to be covered, and it took weeks before the donor sites were healed. Grafting on irregular surfaces (especially bare bone defects) was very difficult. The donor area looked ugly for at least six months. He wondered whether integument could be obtained in a simpler way, e.g. by applying lumps of epithelial tissue which might serve as a centre for further epithelialization (von Mangoldt 1895). Von Mangoldt apparently did not realize that the same question had been raised 20 years earlier, e.g. by Fiddes.

In fact his only concern was whether epithelialization could be promoted; the quality of the cicatrix was apparently less important. He described the results obtained by his "new" method as remarkable. The epithelial lumps, consisting of groups of cells from the stratum corneum, stratum lucidum and stratum basale were obtained as follows: After disinfecting the upper arm, he scraped the skin with a razor until the papillary layer was exposed. The pulp thus obtained was a mixture of epithelial fragments and blood. This pulp was spread on the wound bed with a myrtle-leaf probe or a spatula. The wound was disinfected before the pulp was applied to it. When the wound was covered with granulation tissue, this was scraped off. The blood around the epithelial fragments coagulated quickly and adhered to the wound surface. The wound was dressed with silk taffeta or gutta-percha tissue. After grafting on legs, the limbs were immobilized and elevated. All operations were performed under general anaesthesia. The epithelial particles were not separately distinguishable on the first postoperative day.

The wound bed had a yellowish-grey colour caused by fibrin, which disappeared on the fifth to the seventh day; the wound then seemed covered by a bluish-pink film. After 17 to 21 days the wound was entirely covered by "skin", von Mangoldt maintained. Later, this "skin" thickened and desquamation started, which he ascribed to the absence of glandular tissue. He tried to prevent desquamation by greasing the scar. On the basis of microscopic findings he was unable to identify the epithelial components from which epithelialization started; he assumed that it originated from the cells of the basal layer. He obtained the best results on dry wounds and when taking aseptic precautions. After grafting epithelial pulp, wound healing took 8–10 days longer than after conventional grafting. Von Mangoldt reported the results of "epithelial pulp grafting" in eight patients as good; unfortunately, he did not mention how long the patients had been followed up.

In 1903 von Mangoldt once again raised the subject of his method. In a paper on the repair of bone defects, he suggested using epithelial pulp, stating that this produced results as good as those obtained with split-skin grafts (von Mangoldt 1903).

Mann (1895), who worked in the same hospital as von Mangoldt in Dresden (Germany), used epithelial scrapings on patients who had undergone a radical operation of the middle ear. Granulation tissue and a layer of bone were removed 14 days after the operation, and the resulting defect was filled with epithelial scrapings, which were held in position with the aid of a tampon. The entire defect was covered by epithelium within three weeks.

A few years later, von Mangoldt's method was described once more by Noeske (1906), one of his assistants. The technique proved meanwhile to have been changed somewhat. Scrapings from the horny layer were no longer used. Disinfectants were avoided in view of their toxic effect. After four to five days. Noesske observed bluish-grey spots in the wound area, with a diameter of 1 to 3 mm. These islands then increased in size, probably as a result of mitosis and chemotaxis. The latter was believed to be stimulated by smooth granulation tissue. Noeske reported that the grafted area was no longer covered with dressings, although the epithelialization was then slower.

Epithelialization was believed to be stimulated in a cold environment. In some cases the epithelial scrapings were stored in a physiological saline solution if they could not be applied immediately. Dehydration of epithelial scrapings had to be prevented at all costs, although in von Mangoldt's department it had been discovered that the scrapings retained their vitality after as long as 36 hours' drying! Microscopic examination failed to reveal the subsequent appearance of elastic fibres in the epithelialized defect. Noesske (1906) therefore concluded that only fragments of epidermis were transferred in this type of grafting. Consequently he also considered it proven that epithelialization depended solely on epidermis – a fact which virtually nobody doubted any longer at that time. The epithelial cells formed by the pulp were spherical or polyhedral and had more or less sharp spurs which anchored them to each other and to the granulation tissue. They ultimately formed some kind of papillae which resembled those of normal skin. These papillae were formed wherever there were depressions or invaginations in the granulation tissue. Epithelial cells filled these depressions. The greater the distance of the epithelial cells from the original island of epithelium, the thinner the epithelial layer. Noesske considered grafting of epithelial scrapings to be particularly suitable in the treatment of children with burns, who had only a limited donor area, and in the treatment of bone defects due to osteomyelitis. He did admit that the cicatrix was not very strong and contained no glandular structures.

Epithelial scrapings were hardly used outside Germany, but we found a report by the Dutch surgeon, Schelkly (1896) of the Hague, who described how he applied epithelial scrapings to the donor site of a full-thickness skin graft after primary wound healing had failed.

Epithelial scrapings were never widely used to ensure healing of skin defects; the resulting epithelium proved to be too vulnerable. This technique had the same disadvantages as the "pinch" grafts of Reverdin.

Another attempt to obtain an integument by simple means was that described by the American Lusk (1895). While von Mangoldt's method was reproducible, Lusk's was not, or hardly so. In a man who had sustained burns, Lusk covered the granulating surfaces with blister remnants which had remained in situ in the partial-thickness burns. At the time of grafting they were already four weeks old. He had first cultured the blister remnants and disinfected them in a boric acid solution; Lusk reported that about half were accepted, and that "skin" formed around them. In another patient with an ulcer of the leg, he first produced a blister with the aid of "emplastrum cantharides" [9], whereupon the detached epithelial layer was washed with a boric acid solution and stored for three days in a saline solution.

The blister was then placed on the ulcer, which healed within 17 days. Lusk maintained that his method merited wider use because Thiersch grafting was difficult, and because excision of fragments for grafting often caused wounds of unnecessary depth so that healing of the donor sites took a long time. Of this "method" nothing more was heard.

C. The Full-Thickness Skin Graft

One year before Thiersch (1886) delivered his address to the *Deutsche Gesellschaft für Chirurgie,* von Esmarch had addressed the same association with a paper in which he reported his experiences with full-thickness skin grafting. Von Esmarch had pointed out to his colleagues that this type of skin grafting had

9 Emplastrum cantharidum, made up of 24 parts yellow wax, 24 parts resin, 7 parts sesame oil, 34 parts powder from Spanish flies previously dried with the aid of calcium oxide, and 11 parts venice turpentine.

become popular in surgery of the eyelids, mainly as a result of the efforts of eye surgeons like Wolfe and Zehender. Eye surgeons used full-thickness skin grafts in reconstructing eyelids (see Chap. 3).

Von Esmarch had obtained favourable results with grafts of this type in other applications; so favourable, in fact, that he advised others to make more frequent use of these grafts. He used grafts measuring 3 × 1.5 cm, and always removed the subcutaneous fat. Before applying the grafts to the wound surface, they were cleansed with sublimate solution. He advised that the piece of skin to be excised should be larger than the surface to be covered, because immediately after excision the grafts diminished substantially in size. The grafts were fixed in position with catgut sutures.

Von Esmarch used autografts as well as homografts obtained from amputated limbs. He maintained that the full-thickness skin graft was especially well suited to facial grafting. He did regard the persistent difference in colour as a disadvantage, but reported that this difference disappeared after about four months (von Esmarch 1885). In the discussion after von Esmarch's lecture, von Langenbeck (1885) presented a patient who had received a full-thickness skin graft from which the subcutaneous fat had not been removed. It was not until considerably later, that his technique (leaving the subcutaneous layer intact) received more attention. Von Langenbeck had used the graft on a patient with ectropion of the lower lip as a result of burns. The cicatricial tissue was excised, and the graft was used to fill the defect, thus achieving permanent correction of the deformity.

The fact that such surgeons as Thiersch, von Esmarch and von Langenbeck discussed skin transplantation for the *Deutsche Gesellschaft für Chirurgie* illustrates the great interest in this subject. Particularly in English-speaking countries, the full-thickness skin graft became known as "Wolfe graft". Hahn (1888) introduced the term "Wolfe graft" in Germany.

In 1893, Fedor Krause, chief of the surgical department of the *Städtischen Krankenhäuser* in Altona, gave a lecture at a meeting of the *Deutsche Gesellschaft für Chirurgie* in which he reported his experience with very large full-thickness skin grafts over a two-year period (Krause 1893). In German-speaking countries, the full-thickness skin graft is often referred to as the "Krause graft". The term "Wolfe-Krause graft" is sometimes also used (Robinson 1908).

Indications

Advocates of the full-thickness skin grafts recommended many indications for its use. Some surgeons, e.g. Hahn (1888), maintained that the full-thickness skin grafts could be used for all skin defects which required grafting. The French surgeons le Fort (1888), Segond (1889), le Dentu (1889) and Peyrot (1889) urged the use of these grafts on a larger scale because they produced a much better scar than split-skin grafts.

With reference to Hahn's doctoral thesis in Kiel, Wolfe (1889) advocated the use of full-thickness skin grafts also outside the field of ophthalmology. The advocates of the full-thickness skin grafts were of the unanimous opinion that they produced scars of excellent quality (although inferior to the quality of normal skin).

One of the major disadvantages of split-skin grafting was that much contraction occurred. After full-thickness skin grafting this was much less (Watson Cheyne 1890).

Not all surgeons used full-thickness skin grafts indiscriminately. Ceci (1892) and Schelkly (1896) used these grafts selectively, and thought them suitable in particular for corrective and reconstructive surgery of the face. Krause (1893, 1895, 1896) used them mainly in ulcers of the leg. In Krause's department (1890) full-thickness skin grafts were used more frequently than split-skin grafts! The grafts could be applied to muscle tissue, fascia, connective tissue, periosteum, dura mater and even to freshly chiselled cortical bone.

Braun (1899) and Reuter (1899) recommended that full-thickness skin grafts be used only if the integument had to meet high demands. Henle and Wagner (1899) used the grafts not only in treating ulcers of the leg, but also for skin defects resulting from accidents, after tumour excision, in correction of contractures and to replace hairy skin. The results in the treatment of ulcers of the leg were so disappointing that they discontinued the use of full-thickness skin grafts in these cases. The range of indications gradually diminished, but full-thickness skin grafts remained the first choice in the treatment of defects of the fingertips (as a result of accidents, for example) and facial skin defects. Chaussy (1907) was one of the few who continued to plead for full thickness skin grafts in the treatment of patients with ulcers of the lower leg.

Preparations

Antisepsis and asepsis received more emphasis than in split-skin grafting. One of the reasons for this may have been that the full-thickness skin graft became popular somewhat later, when asepsis and antisepsis were already used more widely. Hahn (1888), who worked in von Esmarch's department in Kiel, applied antiseptics such as sublimate or boric acid solutions to the donor site. Watson Cheyne (1890) carefully prepared the area of operation. He scrubbed the vicinity of the skin defect with a strong carbolic acid (phenol) and sublimate solution, and rinsed the defect itself with a zinc chloride solution before powdering it with iodoform. Gauzes soaked in a boric acid or sublimate solution were then placed on the area and left in situ for two or three days. The wound was thus rendered "aseptic" in 24–48 hours and recovered from the caustic consequences of the use of such strong antiseptics.

Krause (1893) performed his operations under aseptic precautions. He prepared the donor site and the wounds with a sublimate solution, and then washed them with saline solutions. The aseptic precautions taken by Henle and Wagner (1899) were described by them in detail: the surgeon's hands and the field of operation were washed with warm water and soap. Disinfection with alcohol then followed. Initially, sublimate solutions (0.1%) and a Lysol solution (1%) had been used as disinfectants, but they were abandoned in view of the toxic effects. During the operation the surgeons wore woven gloves.

Selection of the Donor Site

Although after 1886 skin from the patient himself was used as a rule, this rule was less strictly applied than in split-skin grafting. Hahn (1888), for example, also took skin from amputated limbs or from cadavers. Although Krause (1893) initially stated that he only used skin from the patient himself, usually taken from the thigh, the upper arm or even the trunk, he reported in 1896 that he sometimes used homografts. Henle and Wagner (1899) usually cut grafts from the anterior aspect of the thigh.

Preparation of the Field of Operation

In full-thickness skin grafting, too, the question whether the granulation tissue should or should not be removed was debated. Another controversial point was whether the results of grafting on a fresh surface were better than those of grafting on granulating wounds.

Watson Cheyne (1890) maintained that although grafts could be applied to fresh wounds, granulating surfaces were to be preferred. He regarded the onset of epithelialization along the wound edges as the time of choice for grafting. The period of six weeks initially recommended by Thiersch was too long in his opinion. He did remove the granulation tissue because this gave a smooth wound surface and prevented formation of connective tissue beneath the graft. The Italian surgeon from Genoa, Ceci (1892), who used grafts mainly in reconstructive surgery of the face, did not apply them immediately after creating the skin defects but waited two or three days.

Krause (1893) thought it mattered little whether the wound was fresh or contained granulation tissue. Nevertheless he always removed the granulation tissue, as well as the indurated areas in the wound floor.

Henle and Wagner (1899) postponed grafting when they observed large blood vessels at the edges of a leg ulcer, or when haemostasis was slow. When tendinous tissue was exposed on the dorsal side of the hand or foot, grafting was also postponed until granulation tissue had formed, which was then removed before the grafts were applied, to make certain that grafting was performed on healthy tissue.

Technique of Obtaining Grafts

The choice of the donor sites for full-thickness skin grafts was much more limited than that for split-skin grafts. As a rule, fusiform or ellipsoid strips of skin were excised, whereupon further processing followed. Hahn (1888), Krause (1893), Henle and Wagner (1899) excised the subcutaneous layer along with the skin. This was probably done for practical reasons (the donor defect was then more easily closed). The subcutaneous tissue was carefully removed from the graft. Hahn even described that the graft could have a thickness of only 1 mm after this procedure. He applied the graft as quickly as possible; only if the wound surface was still bleeding were the skin grafts temporarily stored in a sterile saline solution which had been heated to body temperature.

Watson Cheyne (1890) cut strips of skin with a width of 2.5 cm to any length he desired. He ascertained that the subcutaneous tissue was not excised along with the skin. Unless immediate grafting took place, the grafts were first stored in a boric acid solution at about 37 °C. The ellipsoid skin pieces cut by Krause were considerably larger. They were usually 6–8 cm wide and 20–25 cm long. Wagner excised strips with a width of 7–8 cm and up to 45 cm long, mostly from the upper leg. When he wanted to keep the hairs intact, the subcutaneous tissue near the hair follicles was not removed.

Although Langenbeck had recommended the use of full-thickness skin grafts with subcutaneous adipose tissue in 1885, his method found few advocates. In 1893, Hirschberg, at the same meeting at which Krause gave his lecture, again focused attention on this method. He thought that the rich vascular system in the subcutaneous tissue could be of advantage in grafting. It might accelerate restoration of the circulation. Skin grafts could have even better results if the vascular bed of the graft was in a state of hyperaemia at the time of grafting. Hirschberg thus reverted to the views on skin grafting held in the first part of the 19th century (Bünger 1822).

Before Hirschberg (1893) excised the graft, the donor area was rendered ischaemic. It was beaten with a piece of rubber hose for two or three minutes, whereupon three sides of a square of skin were incised. The future graft was lifted off the underlying structure. A pedicled flap was thus in fact created. The cuff was loosened, and the skin became red and swollen within a few minutes. The erection of the skin papillae was even stiff to the touch. After haemostasis, the base of the skin flap was cut and the graft thus obtained was applied to the wound floor. Hirschberg described four cases in which this procedure had been followed. Only the superficial layer of the grafts became necrotic. The integument ultimately obtained looked like normal skin and its sensibility was intact.

Application of thc Grafts

The grafts were generally fitted to the wound edges as snugly as possible, and sutured with catgut without tension (Hahn 1888). Watson Cheyne (1890) used a slightly different technique: he divided the large strips of skin into many smaller fragments, with a diameter of about 1 cm (half an inch) and applied these fragments to the wound bed in such a way that they nearly touched each other. Cheyne did not explain why he used this mosaic technique, but it seems likely that he did this in order not to impede drainage of wound fluids. Like Cheyne, Ceci (1892), Henle and Wagner (1899) did not suture their grafts. Ceci held that this was unnecessary because the grafts showed sufficient spontaneous adherence to the wound surface. The operations were usually not performed under ischaemia. Krause (1893) did first establish ischaemia, but a thin layer of blood nevertheless always formed beneath the grafts.

Dressing Technique and Postoperative Treatment

The dressing technique did not differ much from that after split-skin grafting. Two layers of dressing were generally applied. The first layer often consisted of silk taffeta, isinglass, or adhesive plaster (Hahn 1888). Watson Cheyne first immersed the silk taffeta in a sublimate and then in a boric acid solution before he applied it. The next layer of dressing, which consisted of lint, was also first immersed in a sublimate solution. Cotton wool soaked in salicylic acid was placed on top, and this in turn was covered with a slightly compressive bandage. Henle and Wagner used only a sterile dressing and adhesive plaster. Krause (1893), Henle and Wagner (1899) used an immobilizing splint after grafting on a limb.

The interval until the first change of dressing varied. Hahn, Watson Cheyne and Krause unwrapped the graft after about three days, and subsequently changed dressings daily. Henle and Wagner generally waited nine or ten days before they exposed the wound. After three days the graft varied in appearance: it might show a white, red or livid colour, in which case it was usually swollen. In some cases, blisters even formed.

After seven or eight days the colour gradually changed to pinkish. This pinkish colour became most apparent when the gray layer of epidermis was removed (this layer always completely detached itself after 14 days). The graft healed in 10–14 days (Watson Cheyne 1890), but did not assume a nearly normal appearance until after four to six weeks. At that time it felt elastic and supple, and could be moved over the underlying structure (Henle and Wagner 1899).

Krause maintained that this was already possible after three weeks. At that time he already observed a thin layer of subcutaneous fat beneath the graft on microscopic examination. The grafted skin contained hairs and sebaceous glands, although the hairs were less numerous than they had previously been at the donor site. Sensibility began to return after about six to eight weeks, beginning at the wound edges.

Hahn and Krause also observed that sensibility was only slowly restored. It returned more quickly in small grafts than in large ones. After grafting on a lower limb, the patient was mobilised very cautiously. After healing, which was expected after about two weeks, the patient continued to be confined to bed for some time. Watson Cheyne prescribed two weeks' bed rest. Krause considered a period of three to six weeks to be the minimum required to achieve a fair degree of stability of the graft. Even then, the patients were not allowed to walk.

This long period of bed rest after grafting may have been one of the reasons why Krause was among the few who could describe good results of grafting in patients with an ulcer of the leg. His follow-ups covered a period of one year, but he did not mention how many relapses occurred. He occasionally observed necrosis of the superficial layer of the grafts, and sometimes even of its entire thickness. In such cases debridement was facilitated as much as possible by means of dressings soaked in 1.5% boric acid and 1.5% carbolic acid (phenol) solutions. If the corium of the graft could be saved, a split-skin graft was subsequently applied to it (Krause 1893; Schelkly 1896).

Reports on cosmetic results were rather disparate. Some authors did not mention the cosmetic results (Krause 1893, 1896). Others expressed themselves very content with the results (Hahn 1888; Ceci 1892). Wagner was rather disappointed with them. He considered it a great disadvantage that the grafts could not be taken from a symmetrical site of the body. But not only the cosmetic results disappointed Wagner; he had many failures in which only part of the graft healed or the entire graft was lost. Particularly in ulcers of the leg, his results were decidedly poor. The full-thickness skin graft demanded much of the vascularization of the wound bed, and poor vascularization was one of the principal causes of failure. Another important cause of failure was accumulation of blood beneath the graft. This was believed to prevent both plasmatic absorption and inoculation of capillaries. It was therefore generally agreed that haemostasis was an important (if not the most important) part of the operation.

Infections frequently occurred in this type of grafting. Hahn ascribed most of the infections, to streptococci [10] and "bacilli". Henle and Wagner regarded "Pyocyaneus bacteria" as the greatest enemies of the graft. As long as "Pyocyaneus bacteria" were cultured, he postponed grafting.

Another disadvantage of the full-thickness skin graft was the unpredictable contraction (although the maximum reduction of the graft's size occurred immediately after its excision from the donor site). According to Krause the contraction which occurred during healing was sometimes so marked that the effect of the operation was destroyed by it.

Grafting Hairy Skin

Full-thickness skin grafts were also used in an effort to restore hair growth at a given site. These attempts had a long history. As early as 1818 Dzondi had tried, after reconstruction of a lower eyelid, to restore the eyelashes with the aid of a pedicled flap. Hairs from the eyelashes of the other eye and from other hairy skin areas were implanted in the reconstructed eyelid. The hairs initially seemed to be accepted, but a number were gradually lost. When the patient left the hospital (after an unspecified time), a few hairs were still attached to the eyelid. Dzondi was unable to report whether these hairs were ultimately accepted because he made no follow-up after discharging this patient (Dzondi 1818).

Under the heading "Hope for bald heads", the American *Medical Record* published a report on the promising results obtained by Morrow (1890) with hairy skin grafts used to restore hair growth at particular sites. He punched specimens of skin with subcutis from the hairy scalp and immediately grafted them on a bald spot. The grafts healed within a week and the hairs continued to grow.

Krause maintained that full-thickness hairy skin grafts could even be used to create new eyebrows. Henle and Wagner (1899) presented three patients in whom this had been tried. One of these patients suffered from abnormal loss of hair, and another had lost part of his hairy scalp when he sustained scalp burns. When the grafts healed, the hairs continued to grow, but were later lost. Ultimately hairs did start to grow in the grafted area. In the third patient, an eyebrow had been partly destroyed by burns. An excellent cosmetic result was obtained with the aid of a hairy skin graft.

Von Hacker (1900) also tried to reconstruct an eyebrow with full-thickness skin grafts from the hairy scalp; this was done after an attempt with a pedicled skin flap had partly failed. The graft healed only partly, and all hairs were ultimately shed.

In a female patient who had lost her scalp in a machine accident, Lotheissen (1906) attempted to reconstruct an eyebrow with the aid of skin from the pubic region. The graft healed but the ultimate result was poor because only a few small hairs remained in situ. Several years later, Lexer (1919) pointed out that "hair

---

10 Streptococci had been discovered four years previously by Rosenbach.

replacement" grafting could only be expected to be successful if only very narrow zones were involved, e.g. eyebrows and eyelashes; he preferred pedicled grafts for all other indications.

Healing of Full-Thickness Skin Grafts

The healing of full-thickness skin grafts was studied in particular by Enderlen (1897), and by Braun (1899). In the following paragraphs the results of the investigations of Enderlen and Braun will be discussed.

Epidermal Changes

The superficial layer of the epidermis began to detach itself within a few days of grafting, and was entirely detached by the sixth to seventh day. Braun (1899) assumed that the epidermal layer detached itself because it had fulfilled its task of preventing dehydration. The first indications that part of the epidermis detached itself became visible in the deeper layer of the epidermis. The nuclei of the epithelial cells in the future plane of separation showed degeneration, while the epithelial cells at a lower level (in the region of the papillary elevations) remained vital. The epithelial cells around the hair papillae and the sweat glands also remained vital as a rule. Formation of new epithelial cells began quickly. Epithelialization started from the wound edges on the second day. The sweat glands and hair follicles also played an important role in epithelialization. According to Enderlen the sweat glands and hair follicles at the centre of the graft often degenerated and showed leucocyte proliferation. The sweat glands and hair follicles at the periphery made an important contribution to epithelialization. There were spaces between the epithelial cells. The epithelial cells produced within the first week of grafting showed a different structure: they were of a cylindrical shape and contained more protoplasm than normal cells. A complete layer of new epithelium was present on the fifth day after grafting. The new layer of epidermis was thinner than that of normal skin. Braun supposed that the thickness and shape of the skin from the donor site played a role in this respect. Some grafts assumed a brown colour as a result of accumulation of pigment in the cells of the basal layer; the cause(s) of this process remained obscure.

Ectodermal Structures

The sweat glands and hair follicles sometimes showed degeneration. Braun assumed that a correlation existed between the survival of these structures and the patient's age or sex. The site at which the grafts had been applied might also play a role. Enderlen maintained that most sweat glands survived grafting. He demonstrated this in biopsy specimens obtained from grafts 50 days after grafting.

Corium

In the corium, symptoms of degeneration were already discernible on the second day after grafting. Part of the nuclei of the connective tissue cells had contracted within two to seven days, and stained dark in the sections. This was particularly apparent in the cells in the superficial and the middle layer of the corium. Infiltration of leucocytes extended into the papillae and the epithelium. The leucocyte count diminished after the partial shedding of the epidermis layer. The thicker the graft, the less easily the cellular elements survived (Enderlen 1897).

More and more fusiform connective tissue cells appeared in the deeper layers of the corium. It was difficult to establish whether they developed at this site or entered via the underlying structure. Within a few days of grafting the connective tissue fibres were swollen and lost their coherent arrangement. Leucocytes accumulated in spaces between the fibres. The amount of highly cellularized young tissue gradually increased. According to Enderlen, most of the connective tissue was lost in grafting, and replaced by new tissue. Krause and Braun believed that the connective tissue remained intact. The degree of degeneration seemed to be related, at least according to Enderlen, to the circulation. Three days after grafting, vital connective tissue nuclei were present between the blood vessels, which could be injected with blue gum without difficulty. Connective tissue not only increased locally but also by proliferation of highly cellularized connective tissue from the wound edges into the graft. The connective tissue structures mainly accompanied the blood vessels and formed broad or narrow zones which divided various structures such as elastic fibres. According to Braun, most elastic fibres remained vital, although there was some evidence of degeneration. A number of elastic fibres seemed to degenerate within the first week of grafting, but the normal morphology was rapidly restored.

According to Braun, muscle cells and nerve tissue also survived grafting. But Enderlen disagreed. He observed degeneration of the elastic fibres after seven days, the smallest fibres degenerating first. All elastic fibres had degenerated after 33 days. Braun maintained that the disappearance of elastic fibres as described by Enderlen was a symptom of disturbed wound healing. Braun still found normal elastic fibres after nine days. After 21 days, the elastic fibres lay along the edges of the graft, curled up into balls. After 27 days, a network of elastic fibres was present which, after 41 days, hardly differed from the normal situation; only the most delicate elastic fibres had not yet recovered.

Three and a half years after the operation it was only in the vicinity of the cicatrix that a few elastic fibres were observed to be packed close together; all other elastic fibres presented a normal appearance. Braun found no microscopic evidence that old fibres had been replaced by new ones. The subcutaneous fat, which had not been removed from the graft, survived grafting. Braun did find that the fat was often infiltrated with blood corpuscles; he ascribed this to the close contact with the layer of coagulated blood on the wound surface. Enderlen found that, after four days, the adipose tissue contained numerous connective tissue cells engaged in active mitosis, especially near the edges of the graft.

Blood Vessels

No blood circulation was demonstrable within the first two days. It was assumed that, until the third day, the nutrition of the graft depended on the "plasmatic circulation"; this was why the graft presented a swollen appearance, even still on the fourth day. According to Braun, the "plasmatic circulation" continued to play a role in the graft nutrition even after restoration of the blood circulation.

The vessels visualized by injection techniques on the third day were numerous and dilatated; and they were in contact with the wound floor. The injected vessels were often damaged. The endothelial nuclei were small and stained dark. The vessels in the deeper part of the graft and at the edges presented a normal appearance. It could not be established whether these were the original vessels of the graft or newly formed structures. Enderlen suspected that nearly all the larger original vessels of the graft were replaced, but Braun was not convinced of this. Nine days after grafting, the capillaries reached the superficial layer of the graft. The circulation was completely restored within 13 days.

Reactions Between Graft and Wound Bed

Between the graft and the wound bed, granulation tissue first formed, which later turned into connective tissue. The amount of cicatricial tissue varied from site to site. The formation of cicatricial tissue was prevented at sites where the graft had been insufficiently immobilized. At a later stage, a layer of subcutaneous fat was formed (sometimes within 16 days). Braun thought that "skin tissue cells" were converted to fat cells. In his opinion, this layer of subcutaneous fat gave the graft its pliancy.

Conclusion

In the final analysis, Braun's and Enderlen's views on the healing of full-thickness skin grafts did not differ very widely. Both maintained that all specific skin components survived grafting. The epithelial components degenerated for the most part, but complete regeneration occurred within a short time. According to Braun, the structures of the corium largely remained intact; according to Enderlen, this was not true, the corium was restored by regeneration.

D. The Use of Homografts and Heterografts After Thiersch's Address (1886)

Homografting

Thiersch had suggested that only autografts should be used in skin grafting. There are sound reasons for assuming that his suggestion was based on the conviction that only autografts healed lastingly (Schöne 1912).

Rathey (1886) regarded Thiersch's advice to use only autografts as one of the most important features of his lecture. He himself had experimented with cadaver skin and skin from amputated limbs, but had always obtained poor results. Other surgeons such as Knauer (1889), who wrote a thesis under the supervision of Schönborn, attached much less importance to Thiersch's advice. They maintained that skin from cadavers or amputated limbs, excised within 12–24 hours of death or amputation, could be used without difficulty. In 1888, Bartens had made the same assertion. He had used full-thickness skin grafts obtained from a cadaver to repair skin defects in a patient with burns (Bartens 1888). Bartens had used grafts with a diameter of 1–2 cm, and he stated that an integument of excellent quality had formed (it is strange that his patient was not discharged from hospital until six months after the operation).

Some surgeons considered neonatal skin to be very suitable as graft material. Ivanova (1890) of St. Petersburg described a case in which full-thickness skin grafts from a newborn child were used. She preferred this skin because she held that its vitality was greater.

In hospitals where autografts were used as a rule, occasional exceptions to this rule were recorded. Hübscher (1889), who described skin grafting results in 40 patients, had used almost exclusively autografts and made an exception only in a few cases, e.g. in the treatment of a one-year-old infant with burns of the buttocks; homografts were applied to the wounds because no autograft material was available. The grafts were reported to have healed.

The only homograft applied by Ceci failed.

In the Netherlands, Vermey (1893) described several attempts with homografts. One was made in the case of an 11-year-old mentally retarded girl with burns of the arm. Skin was obtained from her brother. The grafts remained in situ for 14 days, but then gradually detached themselves; nothing remained of them four to five weeks after the operation. Other attempts with full-thickness skin homografts likewise failed.

Overton (1898) was satisfied with the results he obtained with homografting. However, the competence of his evaluation seems dubious in view of the fact that he also described good results with hen's egg membranes (he did stipulate that only the membranes of freshly laid eggs be used for this purpose!).

Homografting was attempted mostly in patients with large skin defects resulting from burns and scalp injuries. In the 19th century, scalp injuries were common in women who worked in factories, where their hair got caught in rotating machine parts and was torn off along with the skin of the scalp. In all these patients, presented only as case histories, homografting led to disappointing results (Sick 1892; Gross 1895; Bivings 1902; Mellish 1904). These authors therefore advised unanimously against homografting.

Heterografting

Hübscher (1889) used heterografts on two occasions. In one case he used skin from the scrotum of a bull: the graft initially attached itself, but gradually disintegrated completely over a period of three months. In another patient, skin from a two-day-old piglet was used. This was likewise initially accepted, but was gradually lost due to suppuration. Hübscher concluded that heterografts were of no value.

Nagel (1889) and Karewski (1898) agreed with this conclusion. Nagel observed that both homografts and heterografts initially seemed to be accepted but disappeared completely within one to five weeks. Despite several negative experiences, publications reporting favourable results with heterografts continued to appear. Many were case reports, e.g. the one published by van Meter (1890). A boy with burns was treated by grafting skin from young dogs. The granulating defects were covered with skin from hairless "Mexican breed" dogs, and with skin from the boy's parents. The dog skin was reported to have given better results than the skin from the parents (the author unfortunately did not qualify the term "better results"). Miles (1890) also used dog skin. A child with burns received grafts taken from the skin of a seven-day-old greyhound. Homografts were also used. According to Miles, both graft types produced good results, and seven months after the operation the grafted area showed no tendency to contract, although no hair grew on the cicatrix and there was no discernible activity of sweat glands or sebaceous glands. Sensibility in the cicatrix was reported to be entirely normal, and the colour of the graft did not differ from that of adjacent normal skin.

Miles preferred skin from young animals because it should possess what he described as "potentially great developmental power". Prior to Miles and van Meter, Cadogan-Masterman (1888) had also reported favourable experiences with heterografting. He had used full-thickness skin grafts excised from young rabbits. He did not remove the hairs from this skin because the fur spontaneously detached itself one week after the operation. Cadogan-Masterman admittedly did not deal with the question whether the rabbit skin was accepted. He simply assumed that the deeper layer of the graft was "revitalized". He had never observed epithelialization starting from the edges of the graft. He thought that the applied skin graft did not so much itself produce epithelial cells, but merely altered the wound conditions so that granulation cells could be converted to epithelial cells – a theory also advanced by Reverdin (1872).

Besides mammalian skin, skin from other species was also used for grafting. Redard (1888) preferred chicken skin, which he found very pliable and well vascularized. He used this in performing a skin graft on a two-year-old child with burns of the chest. The burns had failed to heal during a period of eight months. Redard grafted fragments of chicken skin with a diameter of 0.5–1 cm and he stated that a zone of skin with a width of 7 cm formed along the wound edges within two months. He assumed that the grafts had formed epithelial islands which served as centres of epithelialization, which ultimately led to the formation of new tissue which was of better quality than normal cicatricial tissue.

Frog skin, too, continued to be used in experiments. Particularly in view of a publication by the dermatologist von Petersen of St. Petersburg (1885), Dubousquet-Laborderie (1886) resorted to frog skin grafting. In a 20-year-old man, a skin defect which persisted five weeks after he sustained a burn of the foot was covered in part with skin from the patient and in part with frog skin. The grafts had a diameter of about 2 cm. The frog skin lost its pigmentation after ten days and assumed the same colour as the human skin. The wound healed completely within a month. The cicatrix produced by the frog skin graft was soft and elastic, whereas that produced by the autograft was harder, more painful and more adherent to the underlying structure. A few months after the operation there was still no hair growth in the grafted area; nor were sweat glands present. Dubousquet-Laborderie, who grafted on granulation tissue, maintained that frog skin stimulated wound healing and caused "embryonic" cells (cells of the granulation tissue) to be converted to epithelial cells. He did not commit himself about the role the graft had played in the healing process.

One year later, Baratoux and Dubousquet-Laborderie (1887) once again discussed their experience with frog skin. In three out of eight patients with burns, the wounds had healed quickly after frog skin grafting. The failures were ascribed to suppuration of the wound, absorption of the grafts, a change of dressing, or the condition of the wound to which the graft had been applied. In one case, the frog skin had not been applied in patches but in the form of the kind of pulp already described by Fiddes (1870) and by von Mangold (1895). In this patient, islands from which epithelialization started formed within five days. Both authors also described good results in patients suffering from ozaena and atrophic rhinitis, associated with ulceration. Tiny fragments of frog skin were applied to these ulcers, whereupon the skin was tamponaded. The mucosa thereupon softened and the ulcers healed. In another patient, with longstanding perforation of an eardrum, the defect was covered with frog skin and healed within three days.

In another case report, Grange (1887) described frog skin grafting in a boy who had sustained several compound fractures in an accident. The skin defects were covered with frog skin, and the grafts "healed" in eight days. Subsequently, cicatrization was uneventful and no trace of frog skin colour was in evidence one month later. One of Grange's colleagues later examined the boy and confirmed that a lasting cure had been achieved. It was not only in France that favourable results with frog skin were published. Watson Cheyne (1890) reported favourable experiences with frog skin in England, as did Fowler (1889) of Brooklyn in the United States. Fowler grafted skin from a caucasian as well as frog skin on a defect in a negro girl. The frog skin lost its colour and became transparent after seven to ten days, and subsequently developed an increasingly close resemblance to caucasian skin. The Swiss surgeon August Reverdin (1892), who was still using the method evolved by his cousin Jaques-Louis, used frog skin as well as small human skin grafts. He was satisfied with the results so obtained. He reported that wounds covered with frog skin healed within ten days, forming a firm, stable cicatrix.

Although several negative as well as positive reports were published on the clinical use frog skin grafts (Franke 1889), few publications discussed laboratory experiments with frog skin. This prompted Beresowsky (1893) to study the healing of frog skin grafts in dogs and guinea pigs. He applied frog skin to a fresh skin defect and observed that, 24 hours later, the graft had attached itself to the wound floor; between graft and wound floor, a layer of exudate formed which consisted of fibrin, leucocytes, monocytes and erythrocytes. Monocytes infiltrated the wound bed and entered the graft after 48 hours. The glandular structures in the graft were filled by degenerated epithelial tissue and leucocytes. In the middle layer of the epidermis there were spaces which contained small monocytes and leucocytes. Beresowsky interpreted these spaces as symptoms of degeneration. Symptoms of degeneration were also observed in the basal layer.

After three to four days, the frog skin lay detached on the granulation tissue. At the periphery of the grafts the pattern of epithelial cells was found to be disturbed by leucocyte infiltration. A layer of monocytes formed between the epidermis and the corium of the graft. The frog skin had completely disappeared eight days after grafting. In no case did Beresowsky observe symptoms of vitality in the frog skin, nor did he find fresh erythrocytes or formation of new blood vessels. He concluded that frog skin only played a passive role and elicited a foreign body reaction.

It is difficult to draw conclusions about the application of frog skin grafts. Watson Cheyne, Fowler and A. Reverdin were reputable surgeons. It seems unlikely that they purposely lied. Probably the optimistic view about frog skin was based on misguided observation.

References

Abbe R (1898) New method of creating a vagina in a case of congenital absence. Med Rec (1866–1922) 54:836–838

Altermatt O (1897) Ein Fall von totaler Skalpierung. Bruns' Beitr Klin Chir 18:765–768

Baratoux, Dubousquet-Laborderie (1887) Greffe animale avec de la peau de grenouille dans les pertes de substance cutanée et muqueuse. Prog Med (Paris) 5:288–290

von Bardeleben A (1895) Karl Thiersch Dtsch Med Wochenschr 21:311–312

Bartens (1888) Transplantation der Haut von einer Leiche. Berl Klin Wochenschr 25:649

Beresowsky S (1893) Ueber die Histologischen Vorgänge bei der Transplantation von Hautstücken auf Thiere einer anderen Species. Beitr Pathol Anat 12:131–138

Bernhard O (1904) Ueber offene Wundbehandlung durch Isolation und Eintrocknung. Muench Med Wochenschr 51:18–23

Bivings WT (1902) Avulsion of the scalp, with report of a case. Philad Med J 9:1020–1023

Braun W (1899) Klinisch-histologische Untersuchungen über die Anheilung ungestielter Hautlappen. Bruns' Beitr Klin Chir 25:211–242

Brewer EP (1882) On the limit of skin-vitality. Med Rec (1866–1922) 21:483

Brohl (1893) Beseitigung der narbigen Syndaktylie mittels Thiersch'scher Transplantationen. Dtsch Med Wochenschr 19:866

Brüning F (1904) Ueber offene Wundbehandlung nach Transplantationen. Zentralbl Chir 31:881–883

Bünger CH (1822) Gelungener Versuch einer Nasenbildung aus einem völlig getrennten Hautstück aus dem Beine. J Chir Augen-Heilk 4:569

Burkhardt L (1905a) Ueber die Lebensdauer und Lebensfähigkeit der Epidermiszellen. Muench Med Wochenschr 52:2251

Burkhardt L (1905b) Experimentelle Studien über Lebensdauer und Lebensfähigkeit der Epidermiszellen Dtsch Z Chir 79:216–259

Cadogan-Masterman GF (1888) Dermepenthesis. Br Med J 1:187

Ceci A (1892) On transplantation of skinflaps from distant parts by Wolfe's (Glasgow) method. Br Med J 1:803–805

Chaussy (1907) Ueber Krauselappen bei Ulcus cruris Muench Med Wochenschr 54:1980

Coombs CP (1876) Cases of skin-grafting. Med Press 21:179–180

Czygan C (1893) Ueber Hauttransplantationen nach Thiersch. Inangural thesis, Liedtke, Universität Königsberg i. Pr.

le Dentu A (1889) Greffes dermo-épidermiques à grands lambeaux (Jalaguier). Bull Soc Chir Paris 15:778

Doering H (1906) Abreissung der Kopfschwarte. Dtsch Med Wochenschr 32:402–403

Dubousquet-Laborderie (1886) Transplantation de la peau de grenouille sur une plaie bourgeonnante de brûlure. Paris Med 11:529–532

Dzondi KH (1818) Bildung eines neuen untern Augenleides aus der Wange. J Pract Arzneyk Wundarzneyk 47:99

Enderlen E (1897) Histologische Untersuchungen über die Einheilung von Pfropfungen nach Thiersch und Krause. Dtsch Z Chir 45:453–505

Enderlen E (1898) Ueber die Anheilung getrockneter und feucht aufbewahrter Hautläppchen. Dtsch Z Chir 48:1–22

Enz E (1905) Zur Überhäutung und Wundbehandlung bei totaler Skalpierung des Kopfes. Korrespbl Schweiz Aerz 35:701–713

von Esmarch F (1885) Hautlappen – Ueberpflanzung. Verh Dtsch Ges Chir 14:107–109

Everbusch O (1887) Ueber die Verwendung von Epidermistransplantationen bei den plastischen Operationen an den Lidern und an der Conjunctiva. Muench Med Wochenschr 23:1–19

Fiddes D (1870) Skin-grafting (letter to the editor) Lancet 2:870

Fowler GR (1889) On the transplantation of large strips of skin for covering extensive granulating surfaces, with report of a case in which human and frog skin were simultaneously used for this purpose. Ann Surg 1889, 9:179–191

Franke F (1889) Ueber Hautüberpflanzung nach Thiersch. Dtsch Med Wochenschr 15:45–47

Gabel B (1888) Ueber Epidermistransplantation. Inaugural thesis, Kgl Universität Erlangen Nischkowsky, Breslau

Garrè C (1889) Ueber die histologischen Vorgänge bei der Anheilung der Thiersch'schen Transplantationen. Bruns' Beitr Klin Chir 4:625–652

Gerok M (1892) Ueber Skalpierung. Bruns' Beitr Klin Chir 9:329–345

Goldmann EE (1894) Ueber das Schicksal der nach dem Verfahren von Thiersch verpflanzten Hautstückchen. Bruns' Beitr Klin Chir 11:229–251

Goldmann EE (1906) Zur offenen Wundbehandlung von Hauttransplantationen. Zentralbl Chir 33:793

Grange E (1887) Observation de greffe animale à l'aide de la peau de grenouille. Union Med Prat Françe 43:721–723

Graser E (1887) Ueber Epidermistransplantation, besonders auf frische Wunden. Muench Med Wochenschr 34:213–215

Gross F (1895) Le scalp et son traitement par les greffes dermo-épidermiques d'Ollier-Thiersch. Sem Med (Paris) 15:221

Guldenarm (1893) Discussion: Thiersch'sche transplantatie (Vermey). (Thiersch grafting) in Dutch. Werk Genootsch Bevord Nat-Geneesk-Heelk Amst 1:88

von Hacker V (1900) Die Verwendung gestielter, mit der Hautseite gegen die Nasenhöhle gekehrter Gesichtslappen zur partiellen Rhinoplastik. Bruns' Beitr Klin Chir 28:516–527

Hahn J (1888) Ueber Transplantation ungestielter Hautlappen nach Wolfe. Inaugural thesis, Kgl Christian-Albrechts Universität in Kiel, Gnevkow und von Gellhorn, Kiel

Heineke H (1906) Skalpierung. Muench Med Wochenschr 53:944

Helferich H (1894) Ueber die Hauttransplantation nach Thiersch. Dtsch Med Wochenschr 20:3–6

Henle A (1898) Transplantation. Dtsch Med Wochenschr [Suppl 24] 24:173

Henle A Wagner H (1899) Klinische und experimentelle Beiträge zur Lehre von der Transplantation ungestielter Hautlappen. Bruns' Beitr Klin Chir 24:615–672

Heydenreich A (1889) Transplantation cutanée par la méthode de Thiersch. Rev Chir (Paris) 9:908–909

Hirschberg M (1893) Ueber die Wiederanheilung vollständig vom Körper getrennter die ganze Fettschicht enthaltender Hautstücke. Verh Dtsch Ges Chir 22:52–63 Zentralbl Chir 20:9

Hübscher C (1889) Beiträge zur Hautverpflanzung nach Thiersch. Bruns' Beitr Klin Chir 4:395–421

Isnardi L (1905) Ueber eine Vereinfachung der Technik der Transplantation nach Thiersch. Zentralbl Chir 32:370–374

Ivanova SS (1890) The transplantation of skin from dead body to granulating surface (Report). Ann Surg 12:354–355

Jaeschke A (1887) Zur chirurgischen Behandlung größerer chronischer Unterschenkelgeschwüre. Dtsch Med Wochenschr 13:748

Jalaguier A (1889) Greffes dermo-épidermiques à grands lambeaux. Bull Soc Chir Paris 15:775–778

Jungengel M (1891) Die Hauttransplantation nach Thiersch. Verh Phys Med Ges Würzb 25:87–150

Jüngst C (1887) Ueber die operative Behandlung der Narbencontracturen der Hand. Dtsch Med Wochenschr 13:929–932

Karewski F (1898) Discussion: Thiersch'schen Transplantation (Köhler). Dtsch Med Wochenschr [Suppl 20] 24: 139–140
Karg (1887) Ueber Hautpigment und Ernährung der Epidermis. Anat Anz 2:377
Karg (1888) Studien über transplantirte Haut. Arch Anat Entwickl Ges 369–406
Karg (1903) Totale Skalpirung geheilt durch Thiersch'sche Hautverpflanzung. Verh Dtsch Ges Chir 32: 152–154
Knauer G (1889) Ueber die Deckung grosser Hautdefekte mittels der Thiersch'schen Transplantationsmethode. Inaugural thesis, Kgl Julius-Maximilians Universität Würzburg, Bonitas-Bauer, Würzburg
Köhler A (1897) Ueber die Transplantation der Ulcera nach Thiersch ohne Entfernung der Granulationen. Dtsch Z Chir 47: 102–106
Köhler A (1898) Thiersch'schen Transplantation. Dtsch Med Wochenschr [Suppl 20] 24: 139–140
König AF (1901) Zur Kenntnis der Dauerresultate nach Hauttransplantation. Inaugural thesis, Kgl Christian-Albrechts Universität Kiel, Peters, Kiel
Korteweg JA (1893) Discussion: Thiersch'sche transplantatie (Vermey). Thiersch transplantation. Werk Genootsch Bevord Nat-Genees-Heelk Amst 1:89
Korteweg JA (1894) Thiersch' transplantaties (Thiersch grafting) in Dutch. Werk Genootsch Bevord Nat- Genees- Heelk Amst [Suppl 2] 1: 139
Korteweg JA (1898) Algemeene Heelkunde (General Surgery) in Dutch. Bohn, Haarlem
Krause F (1893) Ueber die Transplantation grosser ungestielter Hautlappen. Verh Dtsch Ges Chir 22:46–51
Krause F (1895) Ueber die Verwendung grosser ungestielter Hautlappen zu verschiedenen Zwecken. Dtsch Med Wochenschr 21: 163
Krause F (1896) Ueber die Verwendung grosser ungestielter Hautlappen zu plastischen Zwecken. Samml Klin Vortr NF 143:365
Kuhn F (1906) Tüll bei der Transplantation. Muench Med Wochenschr. 53:2533
von Langenbeck BRK (1885) Discussion: Hautlappen-Ueberpflanzung (von Esmarch). Verh Dtsch Ges Chir 14: 109
Lauenstein C (1893) Zur Gewinnung gedoppelter Lappen entfernt von dem Orte der Plastik, mit Krankenvorstellung. Verh Dtsch Ges Chir 22:58–65
Lauenstein C (1904) Zur Technik der Transplantation nach Thiersch. Zentralbl Chir 31: 1009–1012
Le Fort LC (1888) Discussion: greffes cutanées (Berger). Bull Soc Chir Paris 14:50
Lexer E (1919) Die freien Transplantationen, part 1. Enke, Stuttgart
Ljunggren CA (1898) Von der Fähigkeit des Hautepithels, ausserhalb des Organismus sein Leben zu behalten, mit Berücksichtigung der Transplantation. Dtsch Z Chir 47:608–615
Loopuyt J (1903) Demonstratie van twee patiënten, beide wegens uitgebreide brandwonden met huidtransplantatie volgens Thiersch behandeld. (Demonstration of two patients with large burn wounds both treated with Thiersch grafts) in Dutch. Ned Tijdschr Geneesk 39:156
Lotheissen LG (1906) Ueber Skalpierung und ihre plastische Behandlung. Wien Med Wochenschr 56: 1809/1861/1917
Lucas-Championnière J (1888) Discussion: greffes cutanées (Berger). Bull Soc Chir Paris 14:51
Lusk ZJ (1895) A new and original method for skin-grafting. Med Rec (1866–1922) 48:800–803
von Mangoldt F (1895) Die Ueberhäutung von Wundflächen und Wundhöhlen durch Epithelaussaat, eine neue Methode der Transplantation. Dtsch Med Wochenschr 21:798–799
von Mangoldt F (1903) Zur Behandlung von Knochenhöhlen in der Tibia. Langenbecks Arch Klin Chir 69:82–115
Mann (1895) Die von Mangoldt'sche Transplantationsmethode nach Radicaloperationen chronischer Mittelohreiterungen. Dtsch Med Wochenschr 21:800
Marchand F (1901) Der Process der Wundheilung mit Einschluß der Transplantation. Enke, Stuttgart

McBurney C (1890) Experience with skin-grafting after the method of Thiersch. Med Rec (1866–1922) 38:453–456
Meière JE (1893) A case of skin-grafting ten thousand two hundred feet above sea-level. Med Rec (1866–1922) 43:686
Mellish EJ (1904) Total avulsion of the scalp. Ann Surg 40:644–649
van Meter ME (1890) Note on the use of skin from puppies in skin-grafting. Ann Surg 12:136
Miles A (1890) Extensive burn of leg treated by grafting with skin of dog. Lancet 1:594
Miyata T (1908) Beiträge zum Capitel der totalen Scalpirung. Langenbecks Arch Klin Chir 85:962–971
Monod Ch (1888) Greffe épidermique à grands lambeaux. Bull Soc Chir Paris 14:271–274
Morrow PA (1890) Hope for bald heads. Med Rec (1866–1922) 38:468
Nagel O (1889) Ueber die Erfolge der Hauttransplantationen nach Thiersch. Bruns' Beitr Klin Chir 4:321–340
Narath A (1903) Drie patienten met groote huidplastieken na zeer uitgebreide verbranding. (Three patients with large skin grafts after very large burn wounds) in Dutch. Ned Tijdschr Geneeskd 39:653
Noesske K (1906) Klinische und histologische Studien über Hautverpflanzung, besonders über Epithelaussaat. Dtsch Z Chir 83:213–253
Obst C (1894) Beitrag zur Transplantation dicker Hautlappen. Inaugural thesis Friedrich-Wilhelms Universität in Berlin, Hopfer, Berlin
Ollier LXEL (1889) Des greffes autoplastiques. Rev Chir (Paris) 9:910–911
Ollier LXEL (1898a) Des greffes autoplastiques obtenues par la transplantation de larges lambeaux dermiques. CR Acad Sci 126:1252–1255
Ollier LXEL (1989b) Des modifications subies par les lambeaux dermiques dans la greffe autoplastique et des conditions qui favorisent leur accroissement en surface. CR Acad Sci 126:1316–1319
Overton F (1898) Skingrafting by unusual methods. Med Rec (1866–1922) 54:527
von Petersen O (1885) Ueber Transplantation von Froschhaut auf granulirende Wunden des Menschen. St Petersb Med Wochenschr 1885, NF 2:326
Peyrot (1889) Discussion: greffes dermo-épidermiques à grands lambeaux (Jalaguier). Bull Soc Chir Paris 15:778
Plessing E (1888) Hautverpflanzung nach C. Thiersch. Langenbecks Arch Klin Chir 37:53–78
Pozzi S (1888) Discussion: greffe épidermique à grands lambeaux (Monod). Bull Soc Chir Paris 14:272
Raehlmann E (1891) Therapeutische Erfahrungen über Lidhauten-operation, sowie über Haut- und Schleimhauttransplantation am Auge. Dtsch Med Wochenschr 17:4–9
Ranneft SB (1893) Ned Tijdschr Geneesk 29:880
Rathey (1886) Ueber Transplantation von Hautstücken. Dtsch Med Wochenschr 12:452
Redard P (1888) Greffes zooplastiques – greffes avec la peau de poulet. Gaz Med Paris 7:63
Reuter (1899) Beitrag zur Indikation der Ueberpflanzung ungestielter Hautlappen. Muench Med Wochenschr 46:1675
Reverdin A (1876) Ein Fall von Abreissung der Kopfhaut, durch Transplantation geheilt. Dtsch Z Chir 6:418
Reverdin A (1872) Transplantation de peau de grenouille sur des plaies humaines. Arch Med Exp 4:139–147
Reverdin JL (1869) Greffe épidermique. Bull Soc Chir Paris 10:511–515
Riegner O (1893) Ein Fall von totaler Skalpirung, durch Thiersch'sche Hautimplantationen geheilt. Zentralbl Chir 20:1109–1112
Robinson EF (1908) Total avulsion of the scalp. Surg Gynecol Obstet 7:663–666
Rotgans J (1893) Huid-transplantatie. (Skin grafting) in Dutch. Ned Tijdschr Geneesk 29:880
Schelkly (1896) Over huid-transplantatie. (Skin grafting) in Dutch. Ned Tijdschr Geneesk 32:287–291
Schnitzler J, Ewald K (1894) Zur Technik der Hauttransplantation nach Thiersch. Zentralbl Chir 21:148
Schoene G (1912) Die heteroplastische und homöoplastische Transplantation. Springer, Berlin Heidelberg New York

Segond P (1889) Discussion: greffes dermo-épidermiques à grands lambeaux (Jalaguier). Bull Soc Chir Paris 15:778

Sick C (1887) Demonstration eines 20 jährigen Mädchens, das schwere Verbrennungen erlitten und bei welchem die entstandenen ausgedehnten Hautdefekte durch Transplantation nach Thiersch gedeckt wurden. Dtsch Med Wochenschr 13:798

Sick C (1892) Muench Med Wochenschr 39:115

Thierfelder A (1872) Ueber Anheilung transplantirter Hautstücke. Arch Heilk 13:524–531

Thiersch C (1874) Ueber die feineren anatomischen Veränderungen bei Aufheilung von Haut auf Granulationen. Langenbecks Arch Klin Chir 17:318

Thiersch C (1886) Ueber Hautverpflanzung. Verh Dtsch Ges Chir 5:17–19

Thiersch J (1922) Carl Thiersch, sein Leben. Barth, Leipzig

Tilanus jr J (1894) Discussion: Thiersch' transplantaties (Korteweg). (Thiersch grafting) in Dutch. Werk Genootsch Bevord Nat- Genees- Heelk Amst 1:139

Trnka (1893) Ein Beitrag zur Methode der Hauttransplantation nach Thiersch. Wien Med Wochenschr 43:785

Urban G (1892) Ueber die Hautverpflanzung nach Thiersch. Dtsch Z Chir 34:187–237

Vermey AE (1893) Thiersch'sche transplantatie. (Thiersch grafting) in Dutch. Werk Genootsch Bevord Nat- Genees- Heelk Amst 1/85:143

Wagner H (1903) Die Behandlung von granulierenden Hautwunden. Zentralbl Chir 30: 1361–1365

Waljaschko G (1906) Zur Technik der Hauttransplantation nach Thiersch. Muench Med Wochenschr 53:2055

Watson Cheyne W (1890) Skin grafting. Practitioner 44:401–411

Wauer G (1893) Ueber Prophylaxis und Therapie von Narbenkontrakturen. Inaugural thesis, Friedrich-Wilhelms Universität in Berlin

Weischer A (1906) Ueber die Wundbehandlung nach Transplantationen. Zentralbl Chir 33:689–692

Wentscher J (1894) Die Verwendung conservirter Hautlappen bei der Transplantation nach Thiersch. Berl Klin Wochenschr 31:979–981

Wentscher J (1898) Wie lange und unter welchen Umständen bleibt die Lebensfähigkeit der menschlichen Epidermiszellen ausserhalb des Organismus erhalten? Zentralbl Chir 25: 7–8

Wilms M (1901) Studien zur Pathologie der Verbrennung. Die Ursache des Todes nach ausgedehnter Hautverbrennung. Mitt Grenzgeb Med Chir 8:393

Wolfe JR (1889) On Professor von Esmarch's operation for correcting deformities of the face by transplanting skin-flaps from distant parts without pedicles. Br Med J 1:514

Chapter 5
Skin Grafting During the First Three Decades of the 20th Century

The extent to which skin grafting was done shows an unmistakable pendular movement. After Reverdin's first successful graft (1869) came a period of frequent use of grafts. Subsequently, their popularity waned in view of the poor results. In 1886, Thiersch introduced new principles which led to another rise. But again the disappointing results led to a gradual decline. On the one hand the cicatrices were of moderate quality and shrank, giving rise to contractures, but on the other hand the method became discredited through misuse.

In Sonnenburg and Tschmarke's wellknown monograph (1915) *Die Verbrennungen und Erfrierungen,* [1] skin grafts are only casually mentioned in the chapter on the treatment of burns. During the first two decades of the 20th century, skin grafting seemed to be so unpopular that several investigators urged grafting on a larger scale. This was done in 1905 in the United States by Sneve in the widely quoted article "The treatment of burns and skin grafting"; in England by Douglas et al. (1917) in an article entitled "On skin grafting: a plea for its more extensive application"; and in Germany by Holzapfel in an article with the unequivocal title "Mehr Transplantieren" (More grafting), which appeared in 1916. A number of years later Lexer (1925), [2] a celebrated German surgeon, also observed that skin grafting was still not widely done. He remarked: "Epidermis- und besonders Hautverpflanzungen werden noch immer viel zu wenig angewendet." [3]

Skin grafting activity declined all over the world. In a survey of the history of skin grafting in Russia, Dzanelidze (1952) also stated that skin grafts were infrequently used in his country during that period.

Another indication of the reluctance to use skin grafts seems to be an article by Willis (1925), who advocated early excision of burns, within 1–9 days. Skin grafting was not performed until much later, if at all.

In spite of these limited activities, the first few decades of the 20th century showed some important developments in skin grafting, e.g. in the indications for

---

1 "Burns and Frostbite."

2 Lexer is considered to be one of the founders of plastic surgery. He received his surgical training from Bergmann in Berlin. In 1905 he became professor of surgery in Königsberg. Via Jena and Freiburg he was appointed to the chair of surgery in Munich in 1928. He wrote several books: *Die freien Transplantationen* and *Die gesamte Wiederherstellungschirurgie* among others.

3 "Epidermal and skin grafts are still used far too sparingly."

split-skin and full-thickness skin grafting. Studies were made which enhanced the knowledge and understanding of failures of homografting, and new possibilities of grafting were investigated.

A. The Split-Skin Graft

Indications

William S. Halsted [4], Professor of Surgery at the Johns Hopkins Hospital, Baltimore, advocated in 1913 the wider use of split-skin grafts after mammectomy (Halsted 1913). In follow-up studies on patients with mammary tumours, a relation was found between survival and the amount of mammary skin removed along with the tumour. In some cases, an insufficient amount of skin was excised because otherwise the wound could not be closed. In other cases attempts were made to close the skin defect at all costs under severe tension, which gave rise to disturbances in shoulder function.

Halsted maintained that no concessions should be made to the principles of tumour surgery, and that as much skin should be excised as radical tumour excision required. When the wound could not be closed, a skin graft should be applied, either immediately or later. The patients then retained the normal mobility of the shoulder, and the long-term survival chances were better.

In his follow-ups, Halsted noticed several other things. Skin grafts seemed to be a barrier against local metastases. In some cases he saw metastases at the periphery of the cicatrix, but not in the grafted area. Moreover, metastases beneath the graft were detected early.

Full-thickness skin grafts applied to fresh wounds healed well. McWilliams (1924) even estimated that graft healing was 100% certain. Split-skin grafts were applied by this author mainly to non-functional body parts. Full-thickness skin grafts were preferred for sites where contractures might occur (Coller 1925). In cases where this was impossible for whatever reasons, the solution was first to apply a split-skin graft, which was subsequently excised and replaced by a full-thickness graft (Koch 1926; Blair and Brown 1929). Both S. L. Koch, of Chicago, Illinois, who was widely experienced in surgery of the hand, and Blair and Brown (1929), who had experience with large skin defects, maintained that defects should be closed as quickly as possible.

Split-skin grafts were more widely used also in reconstructive surgery. Müller (1912) found them very useful in reconstruction of urethral strictures. The strictured tissue was excised, and the resulting defect immediately closed with the aid of a skin graft. Once the graft had healed, the urethral tube was reconstructed by closing the tissues over a catheter. Müller maintained that recurrence of the stricture did not occur; however, his follow-up on five patients was made too soon after the operation (a few weeks later) to warrant definite conclusions.

One of the major contributions to new ranges of indication was made by the Dutch surgeon Esser (Fig. 21), who had been trained by Narath of Utrecht and

4 Halsted introduced in 1889 a technique of mammectomy which is still widely followed.

who spent most of his life abroad. While he was in Vienna in 1916, Esser described a method of using a skin graft on a mould in order to enlarge various spaces such as the conjunctival sac and the oral cavity (Esser 1916). This method could also be used for grafting on irregulr surfaces, e.g. the external ear and the hard or the soft palate.

The principle of his method was that an impression of the surface to be grafted was made in "dental mass". Once the material had set, it was lined with the thinnest possible split-skin graft, with the cut surface outward. The mould covered with the skin graft was put into place, after which the skin was closed. Later on the mould was removed through another incision. Esser based his method on two principles which in his opinion were essential to adequate healing: equal pressure and total immobilization. This grafting method became known as "epidermic inlay grafting" (Esser 1917 a) in English, and as *"Epitheleinlage"* (Esser 1922) in German. Surprisingly, Moszkowicz working in another hospital in Vienna published also in 1917 an article on the same lines; it showed that in 1916 Moszkowicz had given a lecture on the same subject in Vienna. His aim was the same as Esser's (Fig. 22): to

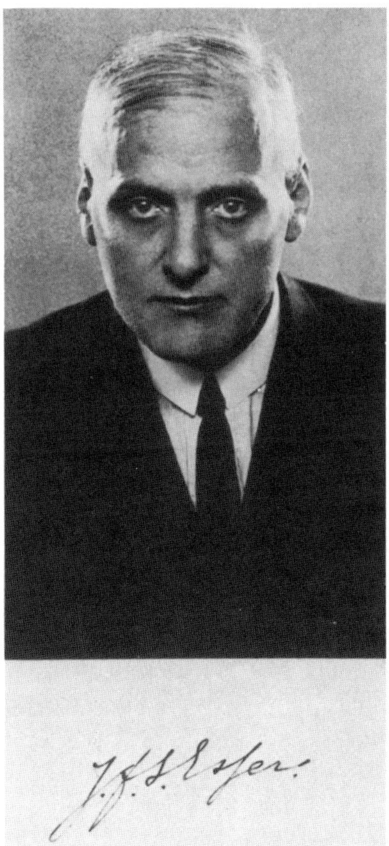

Fig. 21. Johannes F. S. Esser (1878 – 1946), who enlarged the field of application of skin grafts by using "epidermic inlay grafting"

create an epithelium lined space. Moszkowicz did this in the oral cavity, in order to enable his patient to wear dentures. His patient was a soldier who had sustained a severe bullet wound, which had destroyed almost the entire mandible. After wound healing the tongue had adhered to remnants of the floor of the mouth. The patient was seriously handicapped because he could neither speak nor eat. Several operations were performed in an attempt to reconstruct the face. Among other things, a subcutaneous space was created which was later to accommodate the dentures. A graft was inserted into this space in order to line it with epithelium.

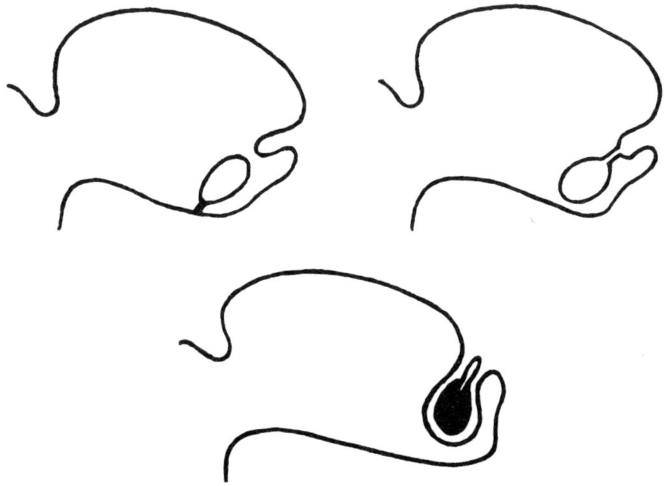

Fig. 22. The principles of "epidermic inlay grafting" presented step by step. The mould covered with a graft will later be removed by an incision in another place (Moszkowicz 1917)

Subsequently the American literature sometimes referred to the Esser-Moszkowicz method (Davis 1917; Douglas 1923).

In 1917 (when Esser was working in Berlin) he suggested a new indication for split-skin grafting, which he had evolved in Professor Verebely's department of surgery in Budapest (Hungary). He had been prompted by serious problems encountered in reconstruction of oesophageal strictures resulting from caustic burns, in which case oesophageal continuity was usually restored by interposing jejunum. The extrathoracic jejunum was covered with double pedicled flaps for this purpose. Esser suggested a simplification of the procedure by using a length of rubber hose to make a tunnel between the cranial segment of the oesophagus and the stomach. The rubber hose was lined with a skin graft, its epidermal surface against the hose. The reconstruction was carried out in several stages (Esser 1917 b).

Esser also made use of skin grafts and a mould in his attempt to solve another serious problem. Since skin proved to be highly resistant to the chemical effects of urine, he believed that skin grafts could be effectively used in patients with exstrophy of the bladder. The reconstruction was of very simple design. An incision was made in the abdominal skin cranial to the bladder remnant. The subcutaneous tissues were undermined as far as the bladder remnant, and "dental mass" was then used to make an impression of the tunnel. The mould was lined with a skin graft; the top surface of the graft was first painted with albumin in order to ensure adequate adhesion to the mould. Mould and graft were then placed in the subcutaneous space and the wound was closed. The mould was removed one or two weeks later. Subsequently, a communication was established between the epithelium-lined space and the bladder remnant. Esser used this procedure in the treatment of three patients. One died of tuberculosis nine days after the operation; the postmortem revealed no signs of nephritis. The other two patients still had fistulae when Esser left Budapest (Esser 1917 c).

Esser's publications attracted the attention of the Gillies group in Sidcup in Kent, England. This group played an active part in the treatment by plastic and reconstructive surgery of soldiers wounded in World War I. The "epithelial inlay" of Esser was used on a large scale.

Without doubt the First World War influenced the development of plastic surgery. Skin grafting was an important part of that branch of surgery. In 1918, at a meeting of the Ophthalmological Society of the United Kingdom, Gillies gave a lecture on the "epithelial inlay" and on a modification of Esser's method: the "epithelial outlay" (Gillies 1918). Gillies had vast experience with the "epithelial inlay", which was used "for ectropion conditions of any mucous orifice, such as turned-out lower eyelids, for increasing the depth of buccal sulci, for enlarging eyesockets, etc.". However, he cautioned against taking the operation too lightly. It had to be performed with painstaking care. For example, when the operation was performed in order to enlarge an eyesocket, an eye prosthesis should be held in readiness before the mould was removed. When the mould was removed, the prosthesis had to be inserted immediately, lest contraction of the eyesocket destroy the effect of the operation.

Gillies developed the so-called "epithelial outlay" for various ectropion conditions. He described the principle as, basically, "the controverse of the inlay". It boiled down to the mould being removed by the same route as it had been inserted. Within a short time, Gillies gained considerable experience with the "epithelial outlay" (Gillies 1920). He used it from the start in the treatment of patients with ectropion of the eyelids, e.g. as a result of burns. He soon extended its use in cases of scars and skin defects of the inner canthus region. The results were satisfactory as long as "the musculature of the eyelids had not been destroyed by fire". The operation was not performed so long as the tissues involved still showed contracting fibrotic changes. Gillies' co-workers Kilner and Jackson (1921) described several new applications of the "epithelial outlay", e.g. in patients in whom the external alveolar sulcus was absent or deficient in depth. They used it not only in patients with injuries but also in excessive absorption of the alveolus and when attempts to fit a denture failed because neither comfort nor utility could be obtained, also in patients with abnormally thick labial frenulums and in patients with a hare-lip, resulting in deficiency of the sulcus above and in front. They used it in patients in whom the internal alveolar surface was defective, e.g. as a result of war injuries, and in cases of trismus "depending upon the presence of scar tissue in the mucosa lining the cheek, after removal of the maxilla". In these patients, a mould with its graft inserted at the end of the operation prevented deformity of the face but was also very efficient in preventing postoperative haemorrhage.

The "epithelial outlay" was even recommended after tonsillectomy because it was assumed that grafting of the raw surface would reduce the period of convalescence, reduce postoperative bleeding, and prevent cicatricial contraction. A few years later, Gillies and Kilner (1929) also suggested the use of the "epithelial outlay" in correction of symblepharon.

Both Esser and the Sidcup group used "dental-impression composition" for the moulds. When warm, this material was malleable and could be given any shape desired. When it cooled it hardened and retained its shape. Later, black gutta-percha also proved to be useful for moulds (Gillies and Kilner 1929).

Grafting Technique

Anaesthesia

Skin grafting was virtually no longer done under general anaesthesia during the first few decades of the 20th century. Since 1899 procaine had been available for local anaesthesia. Local anaesthesia was less cumbersome and safer than general anaesthesia. Joseph [5] (1918) was among the few who did use general anaesthesia, because he did not want to influence graft vitality unfavourably by local anaesthesia. Several authors pointed out that skin grafting could well be done under local anaesthesia, and they used this as an argument in favour of more frequent use of skin grafts. Anaesthesia was effected by local infiltration or regional block (Gould and Archer 1915; Schöne 1915; Archer 1917; Lexer 1919; Schlaepfer 1923; Blair and Brown 1929).

The anaesthetics used were procaine, urea hydrochloride, quinine or even sterile water (Gould and Archer 1915). Schepelmann (1911) and Torrance (1920) froze the donor site with ethyl chloride.

The Donor Site

The thigh was generally preferred as donor site. Coller (1925) explicitly preferred the right thigh, but did not state why. His choice was probably prompted by a remark made by Davis (1919) of the Johns Hopkins Hospital, who had observed that phlebitis frequently developed when the left thigh was used as donor site. This complication did not occur when the right thigh was used. The reason for this distinction remained obscure.

Blair and Brown (1929) tried to avoid taking skin from visible, uncovered areas, especially in girls and babies. They observed that this became more and more difficult because athletes in particular covered ever less of their bodies with clothes.

Esser (1916, 1917 a) used only skin from the inner surface of the upper arm for his "inlay grafts", because this skin was thin and elastic. The donor site was cleansed very carefully in order to remove all skin saprophytes. The dead horny layer was removed, but Esser did not describe how he did this. Others usually prepared the donor site by a very simple procedure: shaving, washing with water

---

5 Jacques Joseph of Berlin was well-known for his skill in reconstructing noses. He even had the nickname "Nasen-Joseph" (nosy Joe).

and soap, and disinfection with alcohol (Koch 1926). Gillies (1918, 1920) and also Kilner and Jackson (1921) used skin from the inner surface of the upper arm for their "epithelial outlay grafts".

Preparation of the Grafted Area

In reconstructive surgery, skin grafting was done only if the vicinity of the field of operation showed no suppurative inflammation. The field of operation was washed and, if normally covered by clothes, painted with picric acid; uncovered areas were twice painted with iodine (Blair and Brown 1929).

Blair and Brown reported in detail on the preparation of the grafting area because they regarded adequate preparation as essential to good results. Soiled wounds were quickly cleansed by frequent mechanical cleansing and with wet absorbent dressings. Blair and Brown were convinced that intensive mechanical cleansing was at least as important as various chemical measures. Application of the right degree of pressure was regarded as another factor in obtaining granulation tissue of the right shape and consistency. All dressings were therefore applied under some compression.

Dakin's solution (0.45%–0.5% sodium hypochlorite), introduced in 1915 by A. Carrel for the irrigation of war wounds, was the agent most widely used in the preparation of wounds (Koch 1926; Blair and Brown 1929). This made it possible to obtain rapidly a red, easily bleeding granulating surface which secreted but little fluid.

Development of Technical Aids and Graft-Cutting Technique

Several ways of facilitating the cutting of grafts were evolved during the first few decades of this century, e.g. by Föderl (1905), Hofmann (1907), Conynham (1913), Finochietto (1922) and Bettman (1927). Föderl designed a grafting knife with a handle which curved up and back so as not to be hampered by body curvatures. A sliding bar was fitted at the rear of the blade, while a bar in front served to tauten the skin.

Hofmann fitted a metal bar in front of the cutting edge of the blade (Fig. 23). The distance between this bar and the blade edge could be adjusted with the aid of screws. This bar had several advantages. It kept the skin flat and prevented cuts of excessive depth and, Hofmann claimed, grafts of any desired thickness could be cut by adjusting the bar.

The knife which the Argentinian Finochietto presented at a meeting of the Association of French Surgeons could also be adjusted to ensure an even graft thickness. Conynham and Bettman suggested complete or partial removal of the teeth of the comb or guard of a so-called safety razor, thus obtaining an inexpensive graft-cutting knife that was easily replaced and could cut grafts of even thickness.

Acting upon the advice of Gillies, Joynt (1928) also designed a hand dermatome (Fig. 24). Before the graft was cut, an incision was made in cutis and subcutis and both were undercut broadly with a special knife. A metal plate was then placed in the cut on which cutis and subcutis could be tautened. The graft was then cut out with a dermatome with a roller guard, whereupon the metal plate was removed and the skin incision sutured.

Joynt died a few months after publishing his report, and in his obituary (1928) it was recalled that he had been one of the first surgeons to develop severe radiodermatitis of the hands. The affection had been so severe that amputation of both hands was contemplated. Finally his hands had been saved and their function restored with the aid of several skin grafts! Flick (1930) described another method to ensure a flat skin surface (Fig. 25). Cranial and caudal to the donor site (usually on the thigh) he subcutaneously inserted a Kirschner wire, perpendicular to the length of the limb. Braces were fitted to the ends of the Kirschner wires, and an assistant tautened the skin by traction on these braces, which greatly facilitated the cutting of the grafts. Several years earlier, Kilner and Jackson (1921) had recommended a "skin fixation apparatus" which enabled the surgeon to cut grafts without assistance: the apparatus was held with one hand while the other hand was used to cut.

Several of these technical aids have been used for a considerable time.

Hagen (1924) was probably the first to design a mechanical dermatome, activated by a flywheel (Fig. 26). He designed the apparatus for the rapid excision of skin grafts of even thickness.

Grafts of varying thickness were cut. Esser (1916, 1917 a) cut the grafts as thin as possible, whereas Blair and Brown cut them as thick as they could. They found it

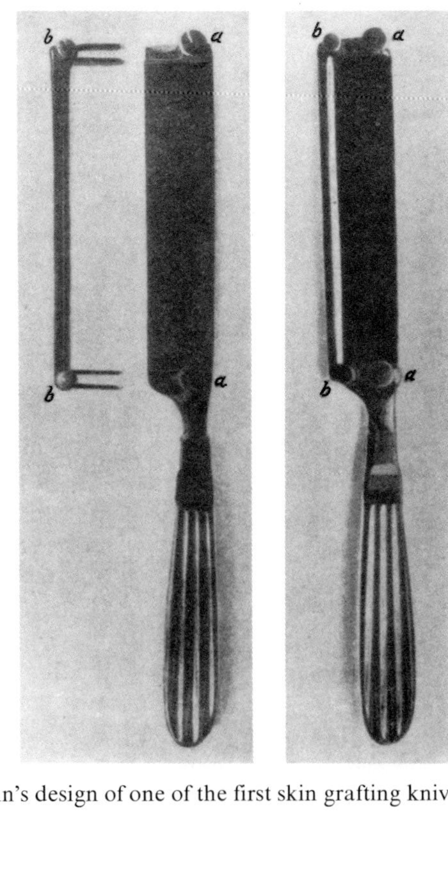

Fig. 23. Hofmann's design of one of the first skin grafting knives (Hofmann 1907)

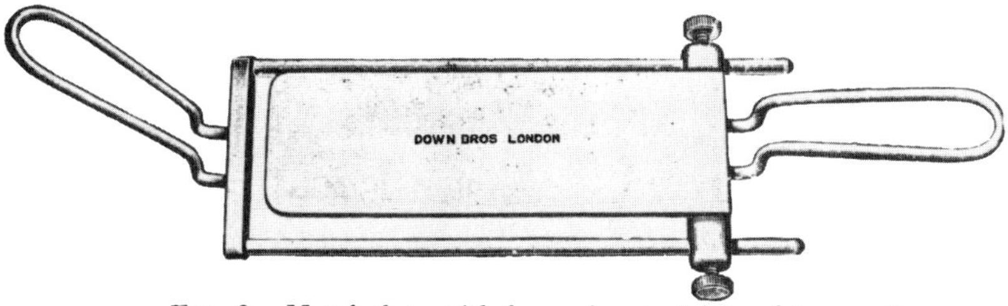

FIG. 2.—Metal plate with frame for stretching skin over it.

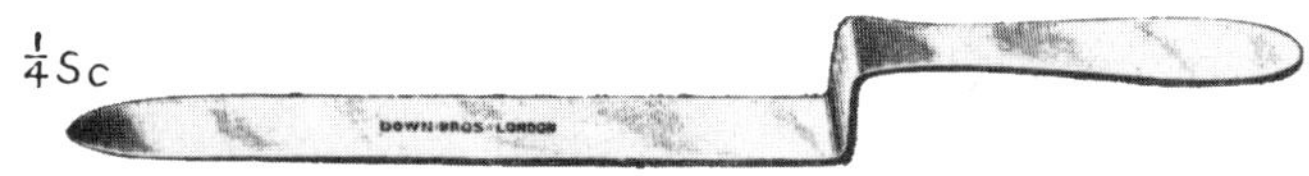

FIG. 3.—Blunt dissector.

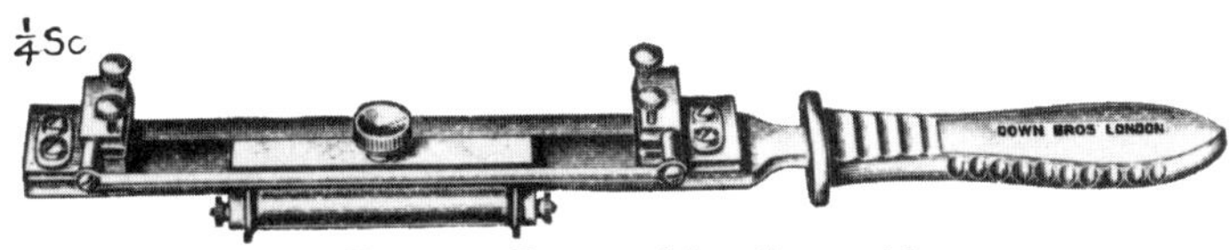

FIG. 4.—Razor with roller guide.

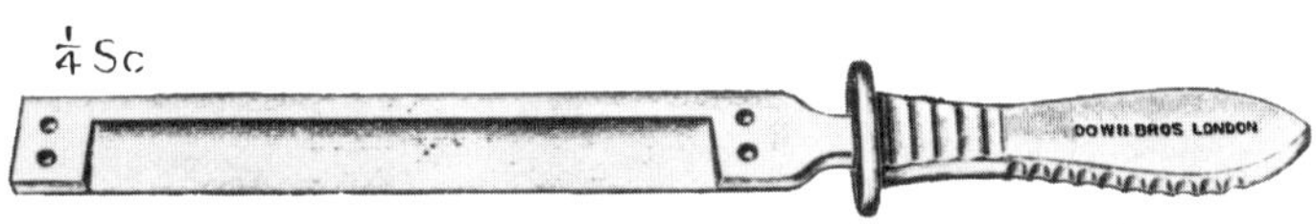

1264/10. Razor with roller removed.

Lane Joynt's Set, for cutting large skin grafts, *stainless steel* (except razor blades), consisting of:—
3 Razors with handles and roller guides, $2\frac{1}{2}$, 3 and 4-in.; Framework to take Rollers; 3 Skin-stretching Frames with plates, 3 widths; 1 Blunt Dissector; Copper Box for sterilizing blades, with handles for lifting out blades, in plain mahogany box

Fig. 24. The skin grafting set designed by Joynt. The metal plate was inserted subcutaneously to flatten the skin (Joynt 1928)

easiest to cut grafts in stout, somewhat obese patients. The cutting was done with a long, light razor, "the skin being held tense and flat by traction pressure of small straight-edged pans above and below the knife". Beside a conventional razor, they also used the specially designed "Blair knife".

In thin patients with flaccid muscles it was much more difficult to tauten the skin properly. "In such patients a suction retractor was almost always necessary to secure the type of graft that was desired." The "suction retractors" were brass boxes, open on one side, which could be connected to a suction system. The open side of the boxes had a number of transverse bars to prevent the graft from being sucked into the box. The boxes were used to achieve a smooth, flat surface and to drain off blood.

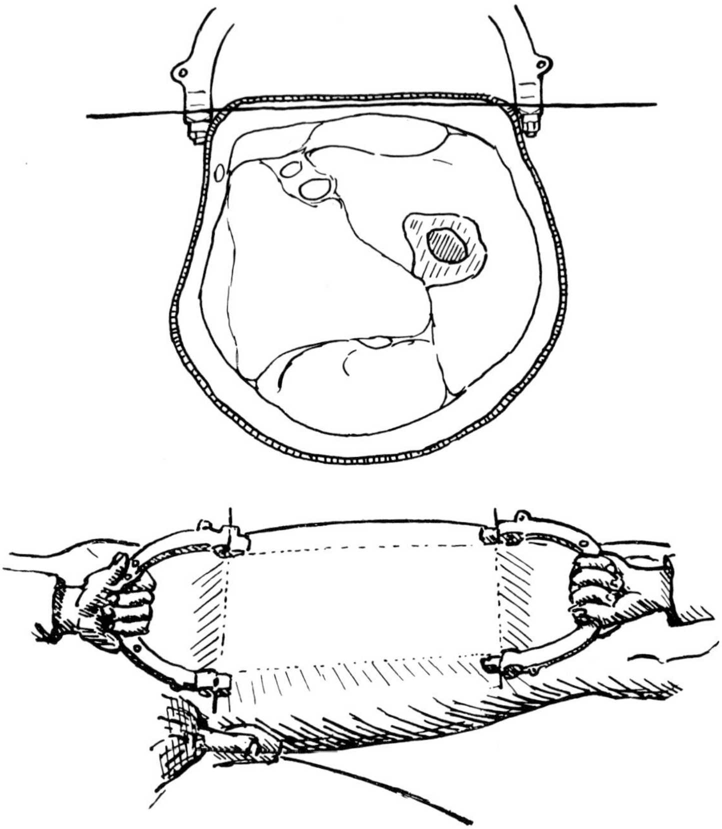

Fig. 25. To facilitate the cutting of grafts, Flick (1930) advised stretching the skin with the help of subcutaneous Kirschner wires

Application of the Graft

One of the most important of the Thiersch principles had been that the granulation tissue had to be removed before grafting. This principle was gradually abandoned, and this may have been one of the causes of the often disappointing results of grafting. Next, the views seemed to change again; several authors advocated excision of granulation tissue (Haberer 1904; Gatch 1911; Enderlen 1912; Coller 1925; Blair and Brown 1929). Koch (1926) of Chicago excised only exuberantly growing granulation tissue.

The graft was often perforated to ensure adequate wound drainage (McWilliams 1924; Blair and Brown 1929). Optimal drainage was undoubtedly ensured by the technique proposed by Lanz (1907, 1908; Figs. 27 and 28), although he himself did not mention this advantage. Lanz had long regretted the fact that, after Thiersch skin grafting, the grafted wound often healed before the donor site did! He therefore tried to develop a method in which not only the skin defect was given a graft, but the donor site as well. He found an ingenious solution when he recalled a children's game: the

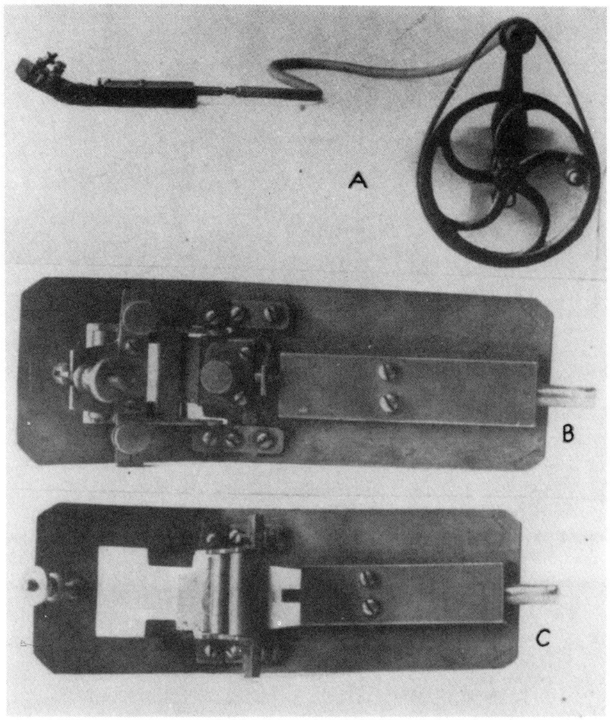

Fig. 26. The first mechanical dermatome was designed by Hagen (1924)

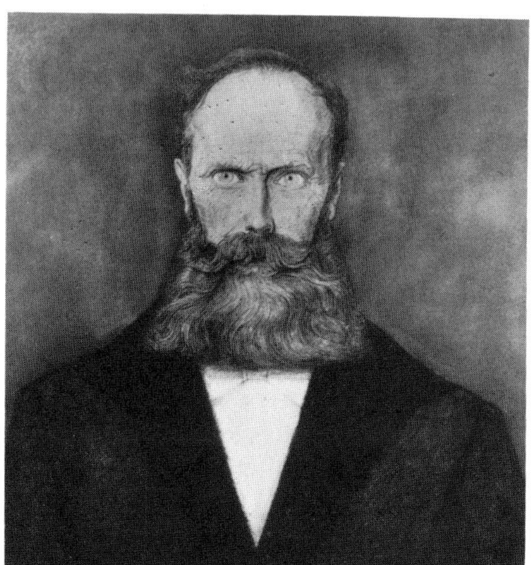

Fig. 27. Otto Lanz (1865 – 1935) from a portrait by the Dutch painter J. Toorop

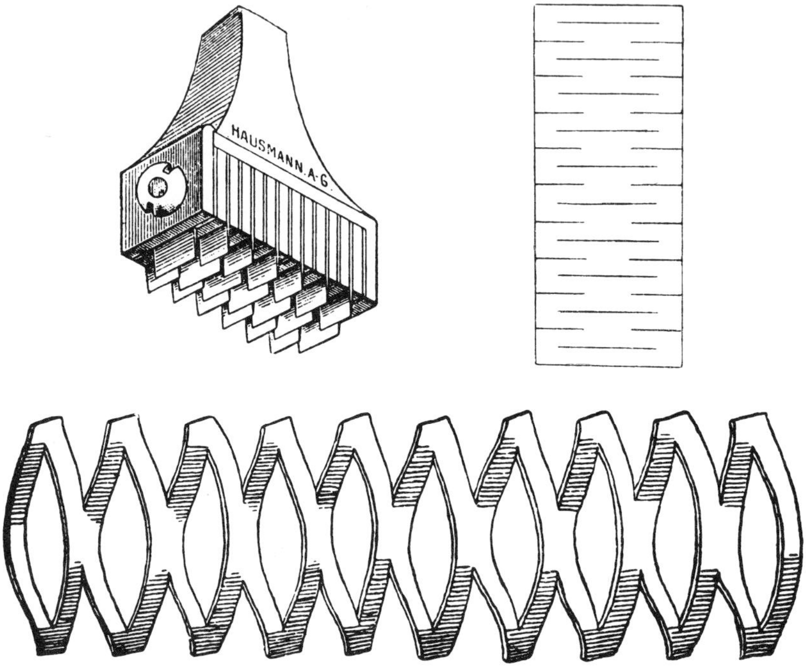

Fig. 28. Lanz designed an apparatus to increase the skin area (Lanz 1907)

making of an "accordion" by making short parallel cuts in paper. He had a die designed with which short parallel cuts could be made in a graft, which could then be stretched to obtain a larger surface area. Half of this graft was applied to the wound, while the other half was used to cover the donor site. Lanz thought that this method could also be used for grafts on larger wounds, when insufficient skin was available for graft material. Lanz's invention elicited few reactions. A number of years later McWilliams (1924) described the "Lanz accordion modification of the Thiersch grafts (as) very useful".

The graft was sometimes sutured in position to ensure the proper tension. Blair and Brown used a continuous horsehair suture for this purpose. If at all possible, Esser (1916) used a single piece of skin for his inlay graft. The graft was so cut that the entire mould could be covered. In some cases the mould was first painted with chicken albumin to ensure optimal fixation of the graft, which was placed on the mould and smoothed out as snugly as possible. Mould and graft were placed in the defect, and skin or mucosa was closed over it under tension, with wide-purchase sutures to prevent tears. The mould was left in situ for at least two weeks, and sometimes longer. Blair and Brown (1929), who adopted Esser's technique, used "wax forms" instead of "dental mass" and obtained results as good as Esser's.

After-Care of the Grafted Area

Davis (1910), who worked for Halsted in the Johns Hopkins Hospital, Baltimore, and McWilliams (1924) probably expressed a generally accepted opinion when they held that fair results could be obtained with virtually any type of dressing, or with open wound management. However, they thought that many complete or partial failures were due to graft displacement or accumulation of fluid beneath the graft. They therefore recommended a dressing which caused sufficient immobilization and permitted drainage. For this purpose Davis (1910) used a loosely woven cotton net with meshes of 1 cm diameter, which after many experiments had proved most satisfactory. Smaller meshes became blocked. Because cotton stuck to the grafts, it was first immersed in a solution of 15–30 parts gutta-percha and 150 parts chloroform. The dressing was kept in a bichloride solution, which was rinsed off with saline solution before the dressing was applied. The first wound inspection was made after 36–72 hours, on which occasion the cotton net was not removed.

Subsequently the wound was covered with silver foil, or open management followed. McWilliams applied silver foil immediately after the operation.

Another type of dressing was advocated especially by Coller (1925) who had tested several dressings over a period of eight years. Paraffin, recommended by Davis in 1917, was ultimately found to be the most suitable dressing after full-thickness skin grafting. This was sprayed on the wound with an atomizer, and overlapping strips of gutta-percha were placed on the paraffin layer. A bandage completed the dressing. Limbs with skin defects covered with grafts were immobilized with splints. After grafting on a fresh wound, the first wound inspection was made after five days; otherwise after three days. When the wound was dry, the same dressing was reapplied; an exudating wound was cleansed with Dakin's solution, and open management followed. According to Coller, the paraffin ensured adequate fixation and pressure and was easily removed.

Koch (1926) and Blair and Brown (1929) dressed the grafted wound with gauze containing 3% Xeroform [6] in petroleum jelly, a gauze padding, and wet or dry marine sponges. These layers were fixed in position with a circular bandage. The first wound dressing was made after five or seven days. A dry wound was again dressed in the same way. An exudating wound with maceration of the graft was inspected daily and cleansed. Open management usually followed after 14–16 days (Koch 1926).

Wydler (1914) advocated the use of cork-paper as dressing; it was porous, pliable and easily sterilized.

In general, surgeons tended to leave the dressings in situ as long as possible after the operation. Rulison (1927) disagreed. He maintained that a large amount of exudate accumulated beneath the dressing, and the risk of failing to diagnose an infection in time was so grave that dressings had to be changed every day. He did not fit the grafts snugly but left a space of 1–2 mm between them for drainage. After grafting, fresh wounds were covered with a smooth, non-adhesive material, strips of thin gutta-percha tissue or plain "cello-silk". The strips, roughly 1 to 1.5 cm in width, were applied in criss-cross fashion. A highly absorbent gauze dressing moistened with boric acid was placed on top. All dressings were carefully removed 24 hours later. The wound surface was cleansed and blisters (if any) were punctured, whereupon another dressing of strips of "cello-silk" and gauze was

6 Bismuth tribromphenate (B.P.C. 1949).

applied. The wound was inspected daily until the fourth or fifth day. Open management then followed.

Besides the surgeons who used dressings on grafted wounds, there were advocates of open management (Wiener 1913; Greenfield 1917; Smythe 1922). After seven or eight days Wiener applied an ichthyol dressing to loosen the crusts. Before the second week he used no wet dressings, lest the grafts degenerated. Smythe (1922) protected the grafted area with a flexible wire splint as a cage.

In 1924, Blair addressed the Illinois State Medical Society with a paper entitled "The influence of mechanical pressure on wound healing". In this paper he took a firm stance against surgeons who believed that aseptic precautions were sufficient to ensure a completely successful skin graft. In his opinion these surgeons ignored a factor of great influence on the result of skin grafting: the pressure applied to the graft. On the basis of clinical observations he had reached the conclusion that sufficient pressure was a much more important factor in the prevention of infection than "the most painstaking attempts at an aseptic technic". He explained the favourable effect of pressure as follows: by properly applied mechanical pressure, dead spaces were eliminated, oozing was controlled, venous and lymph stasis was limited, and the amount of exudate that poured into the wound was reduced.

After-Care of the Donor Site

The donor site was usually dressed in the same way as the grafted wound. The dressing was left in situ somewhat longer and was usually removed after about ten days when the donor site had healed.

Further Investigations into Healing

Microscopic studies of the healing of grafts were also carried out during the first three decades of this century. In Germany, for example, Schöne (1915) resorted to microscopic examination because, for one thing, Davis (1909 b) had postulated that "scarlet red" ointment stimulated epithelialization so that a thicker and stronger cicatrix formed and had therefore advised the application of this ointment to thin, vulnerable cicatrices. Davis came to this conclusion because on microscopic examination he had observed epithelial proliferations in depth at several sites, apart from the thickening of the epithelial layer. Schöne wondered whether such changes had in fact been brought about by the scarlet red ointment. His microscopic study focused on the phenomenon of epithelial proliferations in grafts. Biopsy specimens were taken from grafts applied 5–21 days previously and not treated with scarlet red ointment. Schöne found that, within five days of grafting, there were some sites at which epithelium from the epidermis took a meandering course extending into deeper layers. In some cases the epithelium was even already extending along the undersurface of the corium. Spaces between graft and granulation tissue seemed to be filled by epithelium. Connective tissue formed in the granulation tissue also filled these spaces. During the subsequent days, the epithelial proliferation to the deeper layers of the graft became more and more clearly visible. The strands of epithelium connected with each other. The epithelium proliferated through young connective tissue but never through granulation tissue. After about three weeks, solid strands of epithelium were visible which extended beneath the entire graft. At several sites beneath the graft, at the transition to the wound floor, there were epithelial proliferations which resembled epithelial cysts. These "cysts" contained a central core of keratin and were surrounded by young connective tissue. The epithelial proliferations communicated with the superficial epithelium. Schöne wondered what the cause of this unusual epithelial growth might be. It could not be the scarlet red ointment, because this had not been applied to the grafts studied. The grafts had been applied to a surface of granulation tissue, and Schöne suspected that this was a causative factor (Davis had also grafted on granulation tissue). He believed that the uneven wound surface beneath the graft was levelled by plasma. The several ectodermal structures of the graft, he thought, then formed epithelial off-shoots which filled up the plasma spaces. These epithelial off-shoots connected with each other and fused. The inner epithelial layers keratinized and formed the centre of a cyst. The epithelial proliferations certainly did not originate from epithelial islands which had remained in the wound; nor did they come from two grafts which had been superposed. Schöne believed that the phenomenon of deep epithelial proliferations had no implications.

B. The Full-Thickness Skin Graft

Indications

The full-thickness skin graft gradually came to have its own range of indications, and was used mostly in reconstructive surgery. This was admitted even by Davis (1917), who was a staunch advocate of another grafting technique and wrote: "... Small deep grafts, while more resistant, are also unsatisfactory for the relief of contractures. On the other hand, the graft of whole thickness skin furnishes a most satisfactory solution of the problem ..."

Full-thickness skin grafting produced a cicatrix of good quality which showed no contraction. Not all surgeons thought so. Bier (1918) at that time professor in Berlin, a well-known German surgeon trained by von Esmarch, had so frequently observed disappointing results of full-thickness skin grafting in the course of his training that he advocated the pedicled flap as the only adequate cover for skin defects. The constrictive scars at the donor sites were another serious disadvantage of free full-thickness skin grafts. Bier used these grafts solely on small facial skin defects which could not be repaired with pedicled flaps.

Blair (1924 a), on the other hand, made little use of pedicled flaps because they comprised a redundance of subcutaneous tissue. Full-thickness grafts were applied to defects caused by pedicled flaps.

Operative correction of contractures with full-thickness grafts was most widely performed in patients with scars resulting from burns of the cervical region, axillary region, forearms and hands (Davis 1917; Parce 1922; Blair 1924 a). McWilliams (1924) largely agreed, but added that full-thickness skin grafts were also of importance in the treatment of facial skin defects, and more especially periorbital skin defects. He did not use such grafts on defects in the cervical region, because he found adequate fixation of the grafts impossible there.

The use of full-thickness skin grafts in the correction of contractures of the hand was described in detail by Dowd (1906), Lexer (1919) and Koch (1926), who mostly treated residual lesions after burns. Koch displayed a highly differentiated approach. He applied full-thickness skin grafts to fresh, clean wounds with exposed tendon, bone or nerve tissue, blood vessels or joints. Other factors considered in the graft choice were the size, localization and nature of the wound. If necessary, that is to say if the wound bed was not in optimal condition, Koch first applied a thin skin graft which was later replaced by one that gave a scar of better quality.

Blair described the use of full-thickness skin grafts in correction of syndactyly; Lexer (1919) used them in the treatment of Dupuytren contractures. Dubreuilh and Noël (1911) used them in particular on fresh wounds resulting from tumour excision (surprisingly, especially after excision of tumours from the back of the hand).

Grafting Technique

The Donor Site

Several sites of the body surface could be considered for service as donor site. Davis (1911) held that any part "with sufficient laxity of tissue to admit suturing of the edges of the fresh wound" was suitable. This was very often the abdomen or the thigh (Blair 1924 a; Koch 1926) or even the back (Blair 1924 a) and the trunk (Dubreuilh and Noël 1911).

Smith (1926 a) preferred the inner surface of the upper arm in the male, and the inner surface of the thigh in the female patient, because at these sites the skin was soft and not hairy.

The donor site was generally prepared by washing with water and soap or sponging with ether and alcohol (Davis 1917). Others, like Blair, painted the donor area with picric acid in alcohol.

Graft-Cutting Technique

Davis (1911, 1917) and Lexer (1919) more or less used the technique prescribed by Krause (1893). Both allowed for the fact that the size of an excised piece of skin diminished by about one-third. Both excised an ellipsoid piece of skin because the wound could then be more easily closed after undermining the wound edges. Davis excised skin with a subcutaneous layer. The subcutaneous tissue was removed with scissors, whereupon "leather punch" perforations were cut in the graft to ensure adequate drainage.

Surgeons like Blair (1924 a), Koch (1926) and McWilliams (1926) used a slightly different technique. The contours of the defect were outlined on silver foil, waxed paper or gutta-percha, and the shape of the defect was demarcated at the donor site with a knife. The skin was then excised without subcutis, while Allis or Ochsner clamps were used to keep the skin taut during excision. The subcutaneous fat was removed in a second stage, whereupon the defect at the donor site was sutured. If the defect was too large to close, it was grafted with a partial-thickness graft. Lexer (1919) also did this.

Parce (1922) and Douglas (1923), who cut a full-thickness skin graft in the same way as a split-skin graft, used a safety razor and trimmed the skin fragment to the desired shape afterwards.

Application of the Graft

Davis (1911) also differed from the other authors in applying the grafts to granulating wounds, while virtually all the others applied them to fresh wounds. He initially fitted the grafts as snugly as possible to the wound edges and to each other, without fixation with sutures. Later, Davis (1917) did suture, but without tension. Lexer (1919) likewise held that any tension on the graft was to be avoided.

Other surgeons like Blair (1924 a), McWilliams (1926) and Koch (1926) first attached the grafts with interrupted horsehair sutures, and then ensured good fixation with a continuous suture. The grafts were sutured with some tension in order to keep the capillaries in the grafts open; this was believed to facilitate the "plasmatic circulation". Dubreuilh and Noël (1911) attached the wound edges with horsehair sutures spaced 5–6 mm apart.

Douglas (1923) used adhesive strips with a width of 4 mm for graft fixation. Additional fixation was achieved 12 hours after the operation with a spray of Ambrine or some other paraffin preparation.

Parce (1922) used the same technique as Esser: the grafts were immobilized with a mould (Fig. 29); the graft was tautened with catgut sutures over the mould. Parce held that the combination of tension and pressure promoted healing. Secretion of the wound bed was prevented, the capillaries could heal undisturbed as a result of the good immobilization. Koch (1926) sometimes also used a mould, at sites where he could not apply sufficient pressure by means of a dressing. Blair (1924 a) thought it wrong to combine a full-thickness skin graft with a mould; he held that the mould deprived the graft of the ventilation it needed.

The technical procedure of grafting was generally based on empiricism. Microscopic studies of the healing of full-thickness skin grafts by Davis and Traut (1925) disclosed that there were sound reasons to avoid all tension in suturing grafts (see page 171). Smith (1926 a), Grand Rapids, Michigan, tried to obtain data on the optimal pressure to be applied to a graft. On hypothetical grounds, he was convinced that pressure was important for the healing of a full-thickness skin graft. He regarded a graft as a parasitic object, which depended on tissue fluid for the first few days of survival. Hence the flow of fluid from the wound to the graft had to be optimal in his opinion. Any force which increased intracapillary pressure in the wound bed enhanced the flow of lymph. Since the peripheral venous pressure had long been known to be 5–15 mm Hg, the pressure to be applied had to exceed this value. The pressure in the arterioles was 40–50 mm Hg, and this pressure probably should not be exceeded lest a disturbance in the circulation occur. Smith therefore thought that the optimal pressure should be about 30 mm Hg. His theory was tested in an experimental clinical model; thick-walled inflatable balloons were used to apply a continuous pressure ranging from 30–110 mm Hg to a number of full-thickness skin grafts. Necrosis of the grafts was found to occur at a pressure of 60–110 mm Hg. It was therefore considered proven that a pressure of 30 mm Hg created optimal conditions for healing. Subsequently, Smith (1926 b) designed inflatable rubber balloons of varying size and shape, which could be applied to the

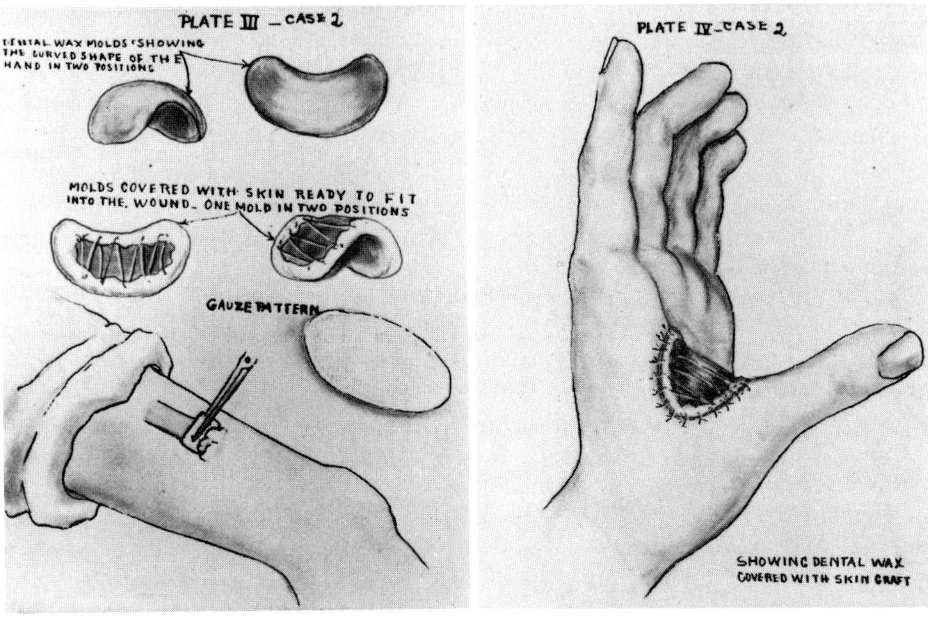

Fig. 29. Parce's technique of graft immobilization (Parce 1922)

grafts beneath the dressing (Fig. 30). Several other surgeons made use of these balloons in their patients (McWilliams 1926).

Davis and Traut introduced in 1926 a modification of the technique of full-thickness skin grafting in order to achieve more relaxation in the grafted area. They advocated this technique for use in areas where the scar tissue was too rigid to shift and where pedicled flaps could not be used. Their technique was as follows. The wound edges of the area to be grafted were undercut over a distance of 0.5–1.5 cm,

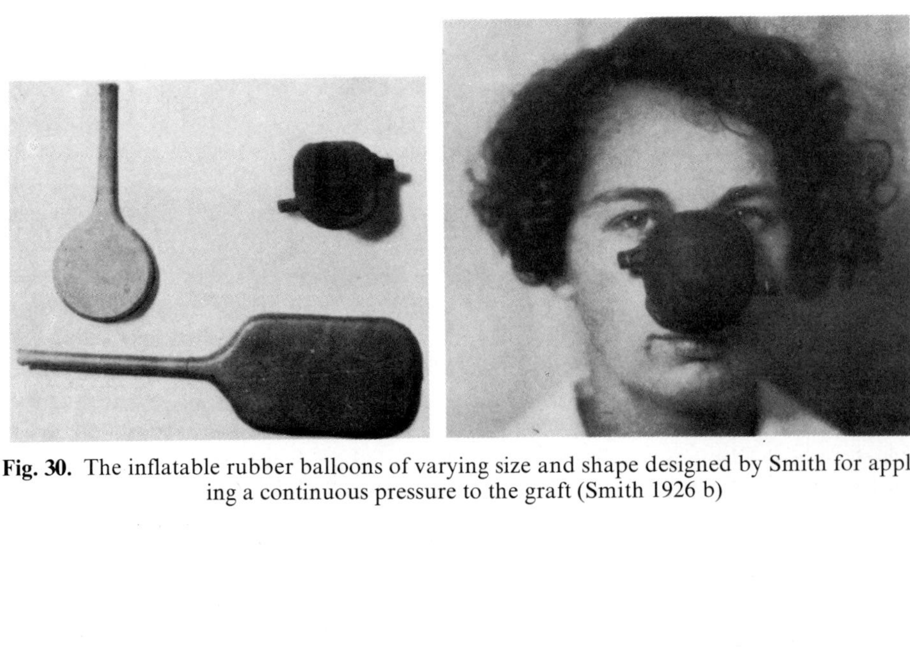

Fig. 30. The inflatable rubber balloons of varying size and shape designed by Smith for applying a continuous pressure to the graft (Smith 1926 b)

and the graft was inserted beneath the undercut edges and fixed with sutures passed through the skin and the graft beneath it. "In the process of healing, epithelium from the edges of the graft and from the scar defect grew toward each other and finally met." The overlapping everted margin was initially rather conspicuous, but in the course of a month or two this margin flattened out and became smooth.

Variants of the Full-Thickness Skin Graft

Douglas (1930) introduced a modification of the full-thickness skin graft: a graft with several perforations which he called a "sieve graft". It was obtained in a rather complicated way: a hollow punch with a diameter of 5 mm was used to punch several holes in the donor area, spaced about 1.5 cm apart. The punch was driven into the skin to a depth of about 0.25 cm. The punched-out pieces were not detached from the underlying structure. A bistoury was then used to cut the skin away from the underlying layer, while the islets of punched-out skin remained in situ. This method yielded a graft with several perforations, and a donor wound with several skin islets. These islets ensured that the donor wound was covered with epithelium in 12–18 days. The perforations in the graft ensured adequate drainage.

Douglas used this graft also on unclean wounds, and obtained a strong scar which showed little tendency to contract. The cosmetic result was poor, and the method was hardly used elsewhere.

Iselin (1916), who worked in Basle (Switzerland) under the supervision of De Quervain, suggested that skin grafts with subcutaneous fat be used, and thus continued in the tradition of von Esmarch and Hirschberg. Iselin used these grafts especially on small skin defects of the fingertips and on skin defects in which tendons were exposed. He considered it hardly a disadvantage that the skin often became necrotic. The fat as a rule survived the operation, and that was what mattered to him. It improved the contours of the fingertips and, because the tendons remained covered with adipose tissue, their amplitude of movement remained undisturbed. The defects later closed by epithelialization from the wound edges.

Nicoladoni (1900), professor in Graz, used an unusual full-thickness skin graft. He grafted a full-thickness skin graft including nailbed and nail, obtained from the second toe, on a fingertip of which all soft tissues had been destroyed (Fig. 31). The graft healed; the nail degenerated but a new nail formed within four months. At that time, protective sensibility had returned but epicritic sensibility was still absent.

After-Care

There was little difference in after-care between full-thickness and partial-thickness skin grafts. Several authors – e.g. Lexer (1919), Blair (1924 a) and Koch (1926) – described the same type of wound management in both cases. The dressings were generally left in situ longer. Koch made the first change of dressing after nine days. Blair inspected the wound after 5–7 days in children, and after 7–9 days in adults. Blair thought it unwise to remove a dressing early, because in that case blisters often formed in the graft, and necrosis not infrequently developed at the blister sites. Blair therefore removed the blisters, if necessary, and painted the underlying tissues with a silver nitrate solution to prevent infection. Necrotic tissue was excised as soon as possible, and a split-skin graft was applied to the defect. Koch likewise occasionally observed small necrotic spots, but in his experience the deeper layers of the skin remained viable and regeneration of the superficial layer took place very rapidly.

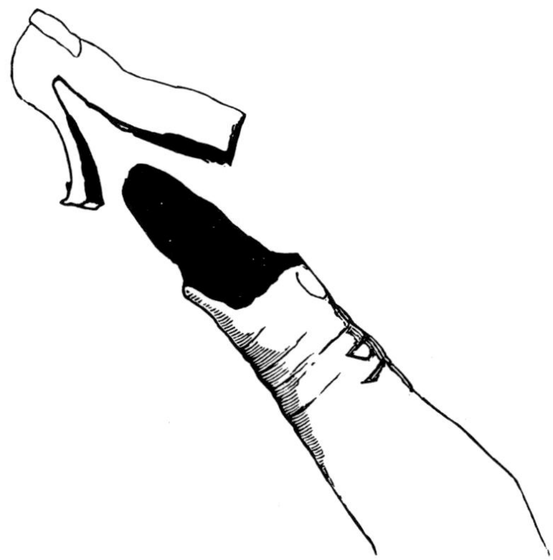

Fig. 31. The composite graft of Nicoladoni (1900); to replace a fingertip, the end of a toe was used

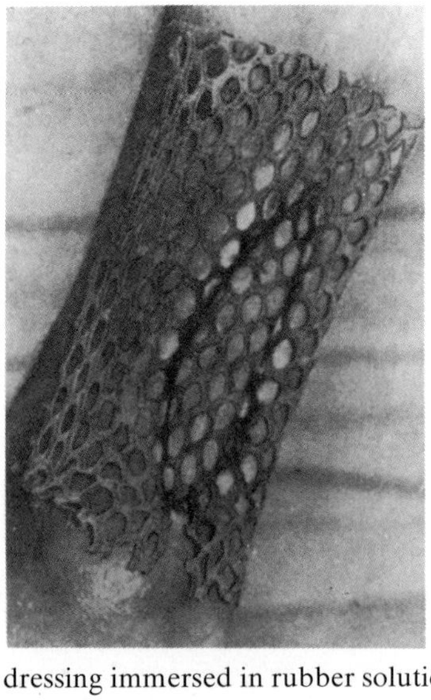

Fig. 32. The cotton mesh dressing immersed in rubber solution used by Davis (1909 a)

Besides silver foil (Lexer) and Xeroform gauze (Blair 1924 a; Koch 1926), rubber was used fairly frequently in dressings because it did not adhere to the wound (Dowd 1906). Dowd placed wet gauze on top of the rubber to prevent it from hardening. He changed the dressing after 8–14 days but left the "rubber tissue" in situ. Grafted hands were immobilized with splints. Davis (1909 a, 1910) initially opted for cotton mesh dressings immersed in rubber solution,[7] covered in turn with wet gauze (Fig. 32). Later (1917) he switched to a flexible paraffin mixture.[8] Parce (1922) who used the mould technique, cut the sutures after 8–10 days and removed the mould, whereupon physiotherapy was usually started.

Results

The full-thickness skin graft was used chiefly in reconstructive surgery, in which restoration of function and appearance should be the principal criteria of evaluation. However, it proved to be difficult to obtain much information on this point. Again and again, evaluation was found to cover almost exclusively short-term results. An exception to this rule was Dowd (1906) (Fig. 33) of New York, who focused mainly on reconstruction of the hands in children and adolescents with defects resulting from burns. In the reconstruction, the defects resulting from excision of the cicatricial tissue were repaired with skin grafts. Dowd extended tendons in the same session. He described his results as observed 4–33 months after the operation. He concluded that, given a wound floor of good quality, the grafts healed well and produced the results desired.

Davis (1917) occasionally observed increased pigmentation in full-thickness skin grafts, although it was less conspicuous than in split-skin grafts. Thick grafts often remained cyanotic in appearance during the first few days after grafting, and sometimes showed irregular contraction. This did not unfavourably influence function.

The results described by Parce (1922) in eight patients treated by the mould technique were so good that he intended to treat more patients in that way. The operations were performed for several different reasons, ranging from contractures of the hands after burns to strictures of the anus.

Douglas (1923) reported on the treatment of burns of the ears. His results were highly satisfactory; infection developed in two of the twelve grafts.

Blair (1924 a) seems to have had the widest experience. He used full-thickness skin grafts on 106 patients: "to release or replace a burn scar" in 57, and "to replace a delayed flap" in 34 (usually on the forehead). Besides the face, the hands were most frequently treated by grafting. Blair attained a 90% result in 58% of his cases. McWilliams (1926) maintained that, given a flawless technique, good results could be obtained in 95% of cases. In his practice, full-thickness skin grafts were used twice as often as split-skin grafts.

Dubreuilh and Noël (1911) noticed that sensibility had not completely recovered as late as two years after the operation.

---

7 Caoutchouc dissolved in chloroform or petroleum ether.

8 Paraffin mixture formula: 18 g paraffin, 6 g beeswax, 2 g castor oil. Sterilized in the autoclave and applied at body heat.

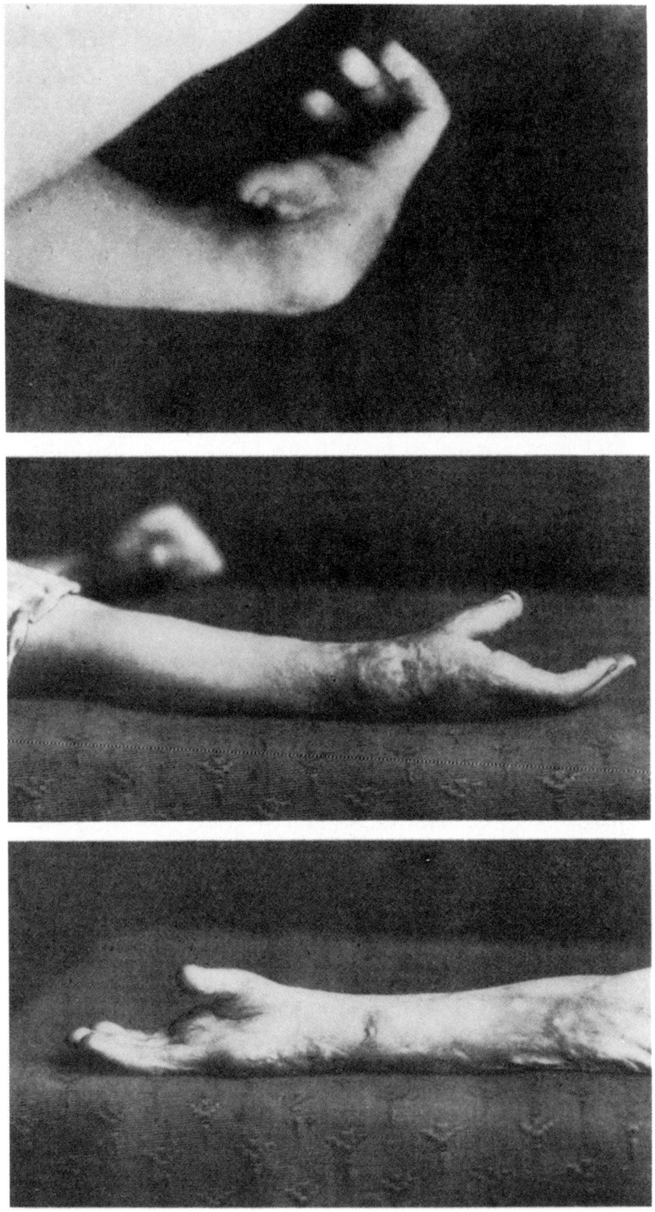

a

b

c

Fig. 33. The deformity in the hand of a young girl one year after a burn injury **(a).** The scar tissue was dissected, after which the defects were filled in with full thickness skin grafts. After a succession of four operations this result **(b, c)** was obtained one and a half years after the first operation (Dowd 1906)

Grafting Hairy Skin

During the first three decades of this century, relatively few grafts seem to have been performed to achieve hair growth on certain parts of the body. Reports on this subject were mostly confined to a few casual remarks in articles on skin grafting, but in the German literature two publications appeared within a short time, with case histories that were more curious than instructive.

In the first of these publications, Lauenstein [9] (1912) expressed his surprise that grafts applied in an effort to achieve hair growth at certain sites ignored the fact that hair roots extended into the corium only in the skin of the scalp, whereas at other places they extended as far as the subcutis. Consequently he wondered whether grafts of hairy scalp skin would give better results than grafts from other sites. He had occasion to test this in practice when a bald patient presented who wished to have hairgrowth on his scalp restored. The patient himself had already found a donor willing to donate a portion of his hairy scalp. Lauenstein then excised from the donor's scalp a piece of skin shaped like a myrtle leaf, measuring 10×5 cm. A piece of the same shape and size was excised from the skin of the recipient's bald scalp, and replaced with the hairy skin graft. The skin excised from the recipient was then applied to the donor site. Prior to the exchange, both grafts were disinfected by immersing them in petrol! Much to Lauenstein's disappointement, the hairy skin graft became completely necrotic. The bald skin graft apparently healed partly. Lauenstein subsequently repeated this experiment on dogs, both with homografts and with autografts, but always without success.

The Russian surgeon Perimoff (1913) described a virtually identical attempt. He excised an ugly bald scar in the temporoparietal region, and repaired the resulting defect with a portion of the hairy scalp skin of a tartar who was prepared to donate this graft at a price of 50 roubles. Perimoff reported that primary healing was achieved in ten days. The hair remained in situ in the graft, and grew well. He assumed that the graft had been completely successful, because he had heard nothing from the patient, who had promised to inform him if something should go wrong! Perimoff maintained that Lauenstein's attempt had failed because he had used petrol as disinfectant. He considered petrol to be toxic. Any doubts about the feasibility of homografting were not expressed in this context.

American journals published several articles on reconstruction of eyebrows with autologous hairy full-thickness skin grafts. Davis (1911, 1919) used "hairy skin from the pubis or any hairy region" for this purpose. He took the direction of hairgrowth into account when applying the grafts. Blair (1924 a) and McWilliams (1926) preferred skin from the hairy scalp because this ensured more satisfactory growth of hair in one direction. The results were rather meagre. In one of McWilliams' patients, the first attempt failed completely but the second succeeded. Blair used eyebrow skin for reconstruction of eyelashes.

Lexer (1919) advised the use of a strip of hairy scalp with a width of 2–3 mm. He used free skin grafts also in reconstruction of eyebrows, but he seemed to prefer

---

9 Lauenstein was a surgeon in Hamburg. His name endures in radiology: one of the X-ray projections of the hip bears his name.

the pedicled flap, particularly since it was usually the upper eyelid that had to be reconstructed (most of these operations were performed on patients with burn scars).

Healing of the Full-Thickness Skin Graft

Several Americans studied the histological processes involved in the healing of full-thickness skin grafts (Davis 1917; Davis and Traut 1925; Smith 1926 a). The findings generally did not differ much. Smith examined biopsy specimens taken two to six days after grafting, and found progressive degeneration of the epidermis as far as the stratum lucidum and oedema in the papillary layer. After ten days the epidermis had healed, and intensive proliferation of fibroblasts was observed in the corium. The elastic fibres showed little or no degeneration.

Davis did observe degeneration of the elastic fibres, which were replaced by new ones. Within two or three weeks he found a thin layer of adipose tissue beneath the graft; he attached great importance to this because he believed this made the graft movable in relation to the underlying structure, so that contracture was avoided.

The most important publication on wound healing was that by Davis and Traut, who studied the restoration of the circulation in the graft. They found that within the first 24 hours, important processes took place in the graft. Monocytes migrated to the fibrin layer between graft and wound floor; next, they entered the corium and the blood vessels of the graft. This monocyte migration was associated with plasma imbibition. In full-thickness skin grafts, it was of paramount importance that the blood vessels be patent, for the "plasmatic circulation" and monocyte infiltration took place via this route. Subsequently the connective tissue structures and the blood vessels in the corium degenerated. The vascular endothelium became almost totally necrotic. A balance between degeneration and regeneration was struck after 7–8 days, and from that time on regeneration exceeded degeneration. The hair follicles and sebaceous glands showed little evidence of degeneration. The circulation was meanwhile restored, three factors playing a role in this respect. The first, earliest communication between these vessels of the granulation tissue and those of the graft was established by anastomosis; the vessels of the graft and the wound bed just happened to touch each other; this happened within 22 hours. The second mechanism of circulatory restoration lay in the growth of capillaries from the granulation tissue; these capillaries invaded the connective tissue of the corium in a meandering course, between the 4th and the 12th days. They had almost reached the Malpighian layer on the 12th day, at which time the capillaries in the graft greatly outnumbered those in normal skin. Later, several capillaries degenerated again. The third contribution to the circulation was made by capillary off-shoots from the granulation tissue, which made contact with the old vessels of the graft. Davis and Traut described such old vessels as having lumina without much resistance, so that the capillary off-shoots could rapidly grow into these old vessels. In some cases an anastomosis developed at the few sites at which the endothelium had remained intact. Since this occurred only incidentally, they regarded it as a factor of no practical importance. Davis and Traut concluded that the second phase (penetration of capillaries) played the principal role in the restoration of the circulation. It was also in this phase that regeneration of the corium started. They thought that their findings had implications for the grafting technique. Any circumstance impeding the inflow of lymph and migration of cells had an unfavourable effect on graft vitality and caused degeneration. Both inflow and migration would be optimal if the graft vessels were open. This is why the subcutaneous fat always had to be removed with a scalpel rather than with scissors (which would contuse the vessels). The tension under which the graft was sutured was equally important because a proper tension ensured vascular patency.

C. New Ways in Grafting, or the Way Back?

After a period of great popularity, the interest taken in split-skin grafting according to Thiersch's principles gradually declined, as has been remarked earlier. The reasons for this decline lay in the poor quality of the scar and the high incidence of infections which caused failures. Another disadvantage was the tendency to contract. Efforts were therefore made to find a safer and better method of grafting.

John Staige Davis (Fig. 34), attracted attention in 1914 with a new technique of applying what he called "small deep grafts". Davis had evidently been looking for a safe, simple grafting method for years; the "small deep graft" was first mentioned in articles he published in 1910 (see page 173). In a later publication he reported that he had been using these grafts since 1909 (Davis 1929).

In evolving his technique, Davis had allowed himself to be inspired by Reverdin's skin grafting technique, as he stated several times. Several authors later

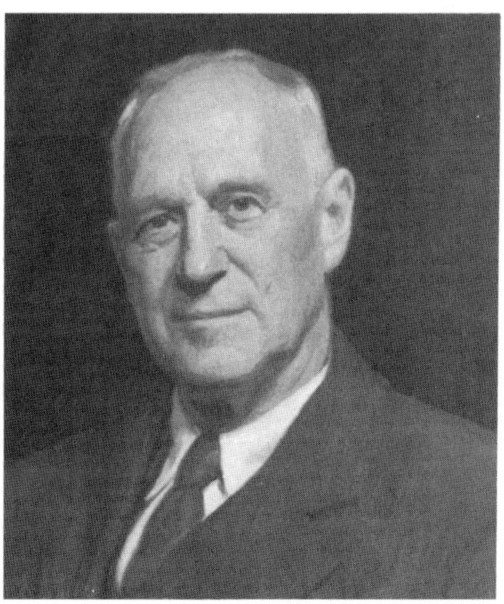

Fig. 34. John Staige Davis (1872 – 1946) from a portrait by Corner. By Davis' efforts skin grafting regained the attention it deserved

remarked that Davis had imitated the Reverdin technique, but in fact there was a difference between Reverdin's and Davis' methods of grafting.

Grafts of this type were described in various ways. For reasons which have remained obscure, the terms used in publications from the Johns Hopkins Hospital varied most widely. Gatch (1911) referred to "pinch grafts"; Reid (1922) wrote about "large Reverdin grafts" and Schlaepfer (1923) wrote about "Reverdin-Halsted grafts". The grafting technique advocated by Davis repopularized skin grafting, as demonstrated by Cassegrain (1924), who wrote:

> ... Up to the fall of 1920 skin grafting was to me a very distasteful operation, necessary at times, it is true, but done always with a feeling of pessimism as to results which was all too often justified. About that time John Staige Davis described a graft which he called the small deep graft. ... I have come to look forward with pleasure to an opportunity of performing this operation.

In England, the disappointing results obtained with large skin grafts had caused the operation to be performed less and less often. This is why Douglas et al. (1917) also tried to evolve a safer method. They, too, reverted to a technique which closely resembled Reverdin's. To the method they developed they attached the name of Steele (1870), one of the first surgeons to use skin grafts in England (see Chap. 2). Their arguments in advocating the use of "Steele grafts" were based on the uncertain results of Thiersch grafting, and on the possibility of sparing the patients pain.

In France, Alglave (1907, 1917) – likewise prompted by disappointing results – developed a method which resembled that introduced by Davis. His technique differed only in the application of the grafts: granulation tissue was excised at the sites to which a graft was to be applied. Other French surgeons, Dubreuilh (1919) and Dehelly (1922) adapted Davis' technique as it was.

In Germany, Braun (1920) used another approach in an effort to solve the many problems and improve the poor results of skin grafting. He applied small partial thickness skin grafts with a surface area of a few square millimetres, not by placing them on, but by inserting them into the granulation tissue. A few years later, Reschke (1922) described a method which had been tried several times in the past: the grafting of epithelial scrapings. He called this technique the Pels-Leusden method, after the surgeon who had given him his training. The skin was scraped with a knife held perpendicular to it. The scrapings from the horny layer were wiped away. The scrapings from the deeper layers of epidermis were mixed with blood and serum, and even with papillary layer fragments. The resulting pulpy mass was injected into the granulation tissue with the aid of a syringe with a thick needle (Fig. 35).

Indications for Small Deep Grafts

Although the small deep grafts were suitable for fresh wounds, they were usually applied to granulating skin defects (Davis 1911, 1929; Alglave 1907, 1917; Dubreuilh 1919; Dehelly 1922; Cullen 1924; Cassegrain 1924). Small deep grafts were generally used for the same indications as split-skin grafts, e.g. to accelerate the healing of skin defects resulting from tumour excision and traumatic lesions such as burns. They were also used for non-traumatic defects such as syphilitic ulcers (Cassegrain 1924). Alglave and Dehelly considered skin grafting indicated when "natural" healing was arrested. Dehelly also used small deep grafts when he wanted scars of good quality, e.g. in functionally important areas where contractures had to be avoided, or sites exposed to injuries.

Braun considered his method suitable for wounds in which other techniques were bound to fail due to the poor quality of the granulation tissue. Wangensteen (1930) gave some examples of such a situation: chronic skin defects near a focus of osteomyelitis, chronic pleural empyema and decubitus ulcer. The cosmetic results obtained with small deep grafts were moderate, and they were therefore not used on facial defects. Holman (1925) did use small deep grafts on a defect of the hairy scalp sustained in an accident.

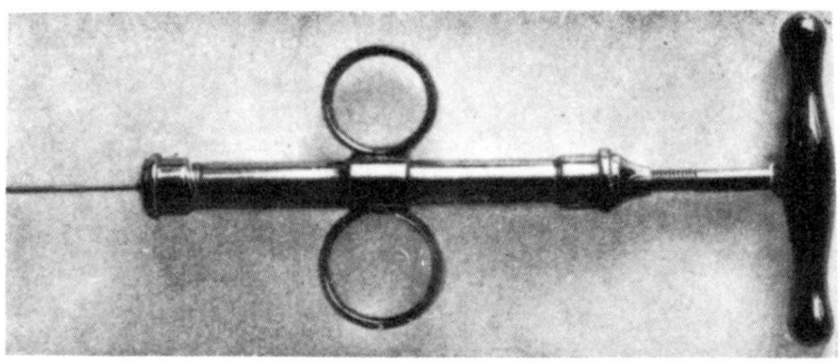

Fig. 35. The syringe with a thick needle used by Reschke to inject the suspension of epidermal scrapings into the granulation tissue (Reschke 1922)

Grafting Technique

Preparation of the Grafted Area

There was no consensus about wound preparation. Davis (1929) even supposed that each surgeon had his own method. Few data were generally given on wound preparation. For small deep grafts, too, granulation tissue was probably chosen that was of firm consistency and showed a "healthy" pinkish colour. In determining the optimal time for grafting, Davis was guided more by the clinical features of the wound than by the results of wound cultures. Douglas et al. (1917) relied more on the results of bacteriological studies. They refrained from grafting when Pyocyaneus bacteria were cultured, because in that case grafting was likely to be unsuccessful. (Meanwhile bacteriological wound smears had become an important part of the diagnostic procedure.)

The wound was cleansed on the day before the operation; secretion and crusts were removed, whereupon the granulation tissue was painted with an iodine solution and the wound dressed with peruvian balsam, castor oil, boric acid or wetted gauze (Davis 1914, 1929). Alcohol dressings were sometimes also used (Cassegrain 1924). Immediately before the operation the wound was washed or rinsed with a warm saline solution.

The Donor Site

Although any part of the body could serve as donor site, the preference was for areas where the skin was not too thick and which were habitually covered by clothing (Davis 1914, 1929; Dehelly 1922). The anterior aspect of the thigh was therefore chosen most often (Schlaepfer 1923; Wangensteen 1930). The donor area was shaved, if necessary, and then washed and rinsed with ether, alcohol or a saline solution (Davis). Wangensteen preferred a more complex procedure and first painted the donor site with iodine, followed by saturated sodium thiosulphate in 7% alcohol.

Anaesthesia

Nearly all these operations were performed under local anaesthesia (Davis 1914, 1929; Douglas et al. 1917; Wehle 1922; Dehelly 1922; Schlaepfer 1923; Cassegrain 1924; Holman 1925; Wangensteen 1930; de Waard 1930), i.e. infiltration or regional block anaesthesia with 0.5% procaine. To Douglas et al. the possibility of operating under local anaesthesia was one of the strongest arguments in favour of a more general use of skin grafts. Only in exceptional cases (e.g. restive children) was the operation performed under general anaesthesia.

Graft-Cutting Technique

Nearly all surgeons cut the grafts in virtually the same way. The operation was performed in bed or on a table, and in some cases the donor area was separately demarcated. Davis used brilliant green for this purpose: the skin was lifted with an intestinal needle held in an arterial clamp, and a skin fragment was cut around the needle with a scalpel. A circular, conical graft was thus obtained (Davis 1914; Dehelly 1922; Reid 1922; Cassegrain 1924; Holman 1925).

Davis (1914) cautioned against the use of scissors which were likely to bruise the graft. A graft cut in the manner described above was not called a pinch graft by Davis, because in his opinion a pinch graft was obtained by lifting the skin with forceps. Alglave too did use forceps to lift the skin in excising grafts. Douglas used a towel clamp for this purpose.

The grafts were always about the same size. Davis initially cut grafts with a diameter of 2–4 mm, but later 4–5 mm. [10]

The reported graft thickness varied. The graft centre was the thickest, and the thickness diminished toward the periphery. In some cases subcutaneous adipose tissue had to be excised from the centre of the graft (Davis 1914; Reid 1922; Cassegrain 1924). At the centre, therefore, the grafts were full-thickness skin grafts.

Schlaepfer (1923), who worked in the Johns Hopkins Hospital, as did Davis and Reid, reported that the grafts he used consisted of epidermis and a superficial layer of corium. Douglas et al. (1917) and Alglave (1917) had previously reported that their grafts had a centre which comprised epidermis and part of the corium. When Dehelly in 1922 addressed the French *Société de Chirurgie* on the small deep

10 The various graft diameters used were about 5 mm (Reid 1922; Dehelly 1922), 6–8 mm (Alglave 1917), 6–12 mm (Douglas et al. 1917) and about 17 mm (Holman 1925).

graft technique of Davis, and indicated that the grafts comprised epidermis and part of the corium, it was remarked in the discussion that the technique therefore did not differ from Reverdin's, because the grafts were as thick as his!

After excision of the grafts, the donor site was covered with a dressing and healing by epithelialization was awaited (this usually occurred within ten days). Only Douglas sutured the defects in the donor area.

Application of the Grafts

The grafts were applied to the wound surface with a needle and firmly pressed in position. It was ensured that the curled-up edges of the graft were carefully smoothed out on the wound bed. The grafts were placed in rows, spaced about 5 mm apart (Davis 1914, 1929; Schlaepfer 1923; Cassegrain 1924). Dehelly considered this distance too large and spaced the grafts only 3 mm apart. Alglave first excised granulation tissue until a bed with a diameter of 8–10 mm was formed, in which the grafts were placed; they were spaced 15 mm apart.

Braun's technique of inserting grafts in granulation tissue, as already referred to above was very simple; Wangensteen (1930) called this method: "tissue culture in vivo". A needle was used to insert the grafts in the granulation tissue to a depth of about 3–4 mm, spaced about 7.5 mm apart (De Waard 1930). The granulation tissue immediately closed around the grafts.

After-Care

The management of the grafted wounds received much attention because the surgeons knew by now from experience that the results largely depended on the quality of after-care. Douglas emphasized that "... the uncertainty of the method is very largely due to imperfections of technique, in particular the technique of the after-treatment".

With this method, too, there were of course different views on the best after-care, and especially on the best dressings. Davis described in detail how he managed the wound. Whenever two or three rows of grafts had been applied, they were fixed in position with rubber strips. The rubber strips were stuck to the skin. Once the entire wound was grafted and covered with rubber strips, wet gauze was placed on top and the patient was confined to bed. The duration of bed rest depended on the site and size of the wound. The first wound inspection followed after two or three days. The wound was rinsed and covered with a bland ointment, or sometimes with scarlet red ointment, petrolatum or zinc oxide ointment to stimulate epithelialization. Hypergranulations were treated with Dakin's solution, but never before the fifth postoperative day, lest the grafts be damaged.

It was kept wet with Locke's solution to inhibit multiplication of bacteria. After skin grafting a limb, the latter was immobilized with plaster of Paris. The first wound inspection took place after one week, whereupon the dressings were changed daily.

Other dressing materials were silk taffeta (Alglave 1917), oiled gaudafil (Braun 1920) and wet gauze (Cassegrain 1924). Cassegrain had the grafted area bathed in warm water from the seventh postoperative day on, to stimulate epithelialization;

others did not follow this example. Why Cassegrain thought that warm water stimulated epithelialization has remained obscure.

A suggestion made by Wehle (1922) did not receive much attention either. He used horsehair sutures "tied around the finger" in a patient in whom a skin defect of a finger had been grafted. In some cases the grafted area was not dressed immediately, but open management was carried out during the first eight hours (Reid 1922; Schlaepfer 1923; Holman 1925). The wounds were then dressed with wet gauze and alternately moistened with saline or Dakin's solution. The latter was used to prevent hypergranulation. Three days after the operation, Holman returned to open management.

After epithelialization of the wound the scar was sometimes massaged to loosen it from the underlying tissue (Alglave 1917; Davis 1929). The troublesome desquamation was treated with a whole range of remedies such as olive oil, theobroma oil, cold cream or some other soothing ointment (Davis 1929).

Results

It was soon found that contraction occurred also after application of small deep grafts. Davis (1914) initially believed that contraction could be prevented by spacing the grafts less far apart, but subsequently (Davis 1929) he admitted that this could not prevent contraction.

The cosmetic results were disappointing. The scar often showed hyperpigmentation, which accentuated its irregular appearance. Apart from contraction, the irregularity of the scar and the hyperpigmentation, Davis also observed keloid formation in some cases. In these patients the grafts lay embedded in the keloid mass. Davis wondered whether a relation existed between grafting and keloid formation, but could not answer this question.

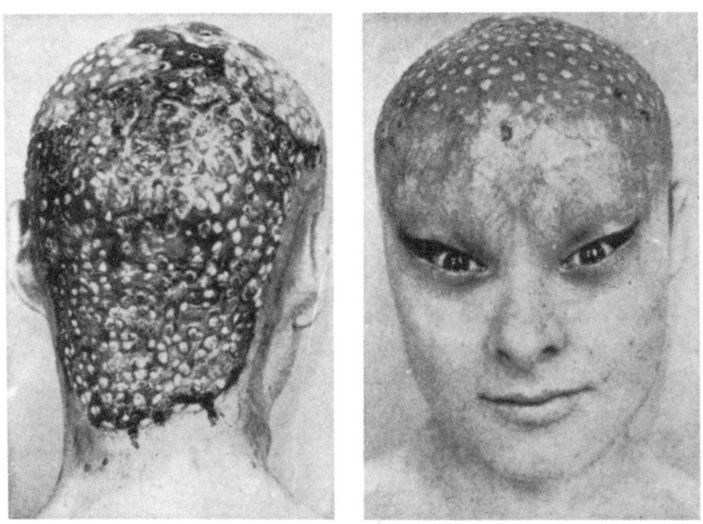

Fig. 36. A patient with a scalp wound. Small deep grafts were applied to stimulate epithelialization (Holman 1925)

Discussions of the results obtained with small deep grafts mentioned very little beyond the fact that the grafts had or had not been accepted. Holman applied no fewer than 809 grafts to a defect of the hairy scalp in a girl (Fig. 36); only 17 degenerated. Cassegrain used small deep grafts on 19 patients, reporting failure in only one patient.

Unlike Davis, Douglas maintained that no contraction occurred after application of small deep grafts; he and his co-workers observed contraction in only one of 33 patients thus treated. Homografts had been used in seven of these 33 cases. The homografts were not mentioned separately but had apparently healed. Although the grafts were still identifiable as such six months after the operation, they described the scars as presenting the appearance of normal skin.

According to Braun (1920) the implantation of grafts also produced fair results: about 50% of the grafts were accepted and epithelialized. No epithelial cysts developed in the granulation tissue. Wangensteen (1930), who used the same technique, was not satisfied with the cosmetic result of the operation. De Waard (1930) of Batavia regarded the thin, vulnerable scar as a disadvantage of the implantation method, and tried to prevent injury by means of protective dressings.

The technique of injecting epithelial pulp was reported to produce the same results as implantation of grafts (Reschke 1922). Reschke even described the scars as thicker than those after conventional split-skin grafting. The scars showed less desquamation and did not adhere to the underlying structure.

The Combination Technique

The technique used by Masson (1918) cannot readily be classified with the known techniques. From a single donor site, he excised a thin split-skin graft, small deep grafts and a corium graft. His description of his technique implies that he must have had great technical skill. With an ordinary razor he first cut from a given skin area a thin graft which consisted almost solely of epidermis. Next, he cut a thin graft from the corium at the same site. If the skin thickness did not permit this, he excised from the corium small grafts which he called "small island grafts". In the third instance, the residual corium was then excised in the same way as a full-thickness skin graft, whereupon the skin defect was sutured.

D. Homografting

Although Thiersch had explicitly refuted homografting and many subsequent publications described disappointing experiences with this type of graft, the first three decades of the 20th century witnessed a continued lively discussion of the possibility or impossibility of homografting. This sometimes inspired rather sarcastic remarks; Holman (1924), for example, wrote: ". . . Iso- or homografting is frequently employed by the profession to the wondering delight of a credulous laity who enjoy contributing small squares of skin as sacrificial offerings on the altar of self-inflicted martyrdom."

About ten years earlier, in a review of the situation of skin grafting at that time, Law (1915) had pointed out that:

> ... A study of various methods of skin grafting has little new to offer, save that two camps have formed, one affirming that homografts do not retain their entity as such, the other believing that nearly 50 per cent of homografts survive. Whichever theory is correct, the fact remains that success from homotransplantation of skin by all of the methods is general, and from the clinical standpoint of results obtained does not differ from those observed in the use of autografts.

Besides surgeons who continued to use homografts as of old (Calot 1913), others distinguished themselves by their efforts to process grafts in a particular way, or because in grafting they took into account blood relationship, age, or blood groups in their efforts to make homografting possible.

Processing of Homografts

Some surgeons processed the graft in a certain way; Gluck, chief of the surgical department at the children's hospital in Berlin for example, treated in 1906 fresh cadaver skin with formalin fumes and with ammonia, in the belief that as a result of this processing the homografts would heal as well as autografts (Gluck 1906). Gluck did not explain why he used formalin and ammonia, and what he expected to achieve. He did not mention permanent healing but referred to the "Type der Heilung unter dem Schorfe" (the type of healing beneath the crust). Krause, who attended Gluck's presentation, remarked that he had never observed permanent healing after homografting. Meyer (1930) later observed that homografts which were immersed in formalin for 24–48 hours loosened after 3–4 weeks whilst epithelialization had taken place beneath them.

A trend in favour of specific preservation of homografts also developed. The skin used was obtained from foetuses which had died during birth. Carrel (1912) played a prominent role in this respect. First he carried out experiments in order to establish whether dog skin, kept in petrolatum at −1 °C to 7 °C for 1–10 days, could be grafted successfully.[11] He concluded that, in dogs, preserved homografts produced "nearly" the same results as fresh autografts, also in the long term. Next, he continued his experiments in a clinical model.

Carrel used foetal skin because he thought its quality superior to that of other cadaver skin. The grafts were first washed in Ringer's solution and then immersed in warm petrolatum. They were stored in a refrigerator at a temperature of 3 °C. The preserved skin was used as grafts in four patients (after 1 day to 7 weeks of storage).

Carrel gained the impression that skin preserved for two weeks was still accepted like normal fresh skin.

In the discussion after Carrel's presentation, Davis remarked that, even without medium, skin could be kept in a refrigerator for a "considerable time". De

---

11 These experiments were part of a far more elaborate study in which several organs were examined.

Martigny (1913) also preserved foetal skin in Ringer's solution but, when storage was to exceed seven days, used petroleum jelly. He preferred preservation of grafts to immediate use because he believed that the preservation stimulated proliferation.

Other Efforts to Ensure Permanent Healing of Homografts

Alglave (1917) believed that skin from relatives afforded the best chance of successful grafting, provided the difference in age between donor and recipient was not too great. He did not specify the observations on which this hypothesis was based.

Inspired by Schöne (1912), who had established that in lower animal species homografting was most likely to succeed between the offspring of the same father and mother, Perthes [12] of Tübingen tried in 1917 to establish whether this rule also applied to human individuals (Perthes 1917). He tested the hypothesis in a 19-year-old girl who had lost her hairy scalp in a machine accident. Autografts were applied to one part of the defect, and homografts obtained from the girl's sister were applied to the other part. Ten days later, all grafts seemed to have been accepted. After four weeks the autografts had formed an epithelial zone, but the homografts had disappeared completely. Perthes concluded that skin grafting between relatives did not lead to permanent healing, and that skin grafting between children of the same sex in the same family could not be compared with autografting.

An article published by the American Masson (1918) revived the interest taken in homografting. He contended that this type of grafting had still not been given the place it merited. In his opinion, the results would be much improved if skin from donors of the same blood group as the recipient was grafted. Given matched blood groups, homografting should produce "nearly" as good results as autografting.

At about the time of publication of Masson's article, Shawan (1919) carried out a detailed study to test this hypothesis. He had noticed that homografts disappeared in a fairly characteristic way: in the course of the second to fourth week, they showed slight desquamation followed by signs of absorption, whereupon they disappeared completely or left only a "bluish pellicle". Shawan wondered whether skin grafting was subject to the same laws as blood transfusion. Shawan's study was interesting in many ways. So far as could be established, he was the first to define exactly what he meant by "primary take" and "primary failure". He was also the first to use the concepts of "biological compatibility" and "biological incompatibility" in the context of skin grafting.

The study covered 26 patients with different blood groups, who received skin grafts from donors with different blood groups. Some grafts were of partial skin thickness and others were full-thickness grafts (which were compared with each other). The grafts were applied in small fragments. The dimensions were not specified.

---

12 Perthes' name is associated with the disease of aseptic necrosis of the epiphysis of the femoral head in children.

Shawan reached the following conclusions: homografts obtained from donors with blood group IV [13] (blood group IV serum agglutinated with corpuscles of groups I, II and III; corpuscles of group IV were not agglutinated by any know serum) became permanent takes and grew almost if not equally as well as autografts. Homografts between donors and recipients of different groups did not remain as permanent growths except when group IV skin was used or when the recipient was a member of group I (serum agglutinated no known corpuscles, corpuscles were agglutinated by serum of groups I, III and IV). Group I recipients grew permanent skin from donors of the four groups. Group IV skin grew permanently on recipients of all groups, but only group IV grafts remained as permanent takes on group IV recipients.

To sum up: "skin grafting obeyed the principle of blood grouping."

It is regrettable that Shawan reached a conclusion within four weeks in all his cases. The patients were usually released after four weeks because the wounds had "healed".

In the experiments of Sokolof (1925) the follow-up period was also restricted to four weeks. Sokolof performed homografting of rabbit skin on rabbits with matched or unmatched blood groups. The best results were obtained in animals with a corresponding "biochemical structure of the blood". Kubányi (1924) came to other conclusions. In his opinion homografts never healed completely but would remain as vital epithelial islands which later became centres of epithelialization.

Masson's publication prompted still other surgeons to investigate the question whether a relation really existed between compatible blood groups and permanent takes (Schlaepfer 1923; McWilliams 1924; (Fig. 37 a–c); Coller 1925; Lexer 1925; Blair and Brown 1929). All of them, however, had to conclude that no permanent healing could be achieved even with blood group compatibility!

On the basis of theoretical considerations, Loeb (1930) considered it unlikely that blood groups could be of importance for homografting results. He maintained that interindividual differences were determined "by all or at least by a large number of genes, while the blood groups depend upon a few genes only. At best these genes, being presumably constituents of the gene set characteristic of the differential, may contribute in a small way to the result of transplantation, but cannot be a decisive factor."

In the Johns Hopkins Hospital, views on homografting seem to have differed for a long time. Gatch (1911) described only disappointing experiences with homografts. Davis (1911, 1914), however, reported good results with homografts. In 1919, Davis wrote in his book *Plastic Surgery* that, on the basis of a retrospective study, he had concluded in 1909 that 40 patients had been successfully treated by homografting in Johns Hopkins. He had to admit that in retrospection the percentage of permanent takes must have been smaller than the hospital notes had suggested.

At that time Davis still accepted Masson's theory that skin from patients of compatible blood groups should give good lasting results, and therefore he continued homografting. In 1929 he wrote that all grafts should of course be taken from the patient's own skin.

Smith (1926 a) obtained favourable results with grafts from donors of a compatible blood group. He even wrote: "It is not only reasonable but highly

13 Shawan used the blood group classification according to Moss (1917), who distinguished four blood groups (I, II, III and IV).

probable that isografts [=homografts] taken from donors with compatible blood types frequently grow as well as autografts, equally certain that such grafts from donors with incompatible blood may grow but will not persist."

This statement is rather strange in view of the fact that Smith in the same article described the histological processes involved in the healing of full-thickness homografts from donors with compatible and incompatible blood groups. Six days after grafting there was an unmistakable difference in histological features. In the graft from the donor with a compatible blood group the epidermis was in good condition. The papillary layer was oedematous, and the connective tissue cells were disappearing. The other graft showed marked maceration and desquamation of epidermis, accumulation of fluid in the deeper layers and loss of staining power of the basal cell layer. In the corium there was marked degeneration with oedema of all structures, invasion with polynuclear cells and lytic changes in the sweat glands.

After ten days the difference between the grafts from the different donors was no longer so marked. After 20 days the epidermis was absent in both, and only occasional corium remnants remained. These remnants were surrounded by granulation tissue which contained phagocytic cells. The descriptions indicated little difference between homografts from compatible and from incompatible donors. But Smith did not discuss this further.

Homografting Tissues Other Than Skin

Besides skin homografting, experiments were performed during this period to study the possibility of accelerating wound healing with the aid of tissues other than skin. In 1913, the American literature almost simultaneously published two articles in which a plea was made for amnion grafting (Sabella 1913; Stern 1913).

Stern regarded attempts to graft amnion as a logical sequel to skin grafting because amnion was also made up of ectodermal elements. He preferred amnion to skin because it was available in abundance. Prior to grafting the amnion was prepared as indicated by Carrel. The membrane was first washed in a saline solution and then dried and kept in petrolatum at temperatures from −1 °C to 7 °C. It could thus be stored for three days. The smooth surface of the amnion was applied to the granulation tissue (the chorionic part thus becoming the superficial layer). The graft was covered with a layer of wax which, together with the chorionic part, was removed two days later (Sabella 1913).

Stern had used amnion grafts on 11 patients, including some with burns. He did not discuss his results in detail. Sabella reported favourable results obtained in five patients, including one with an ulcer of the leg and one with scalds, in whom healing occurred within three weeks.

Gatch (1911) and Davis (1917) had already used the same method in 1909 and 1910, respectively. Their results had been poor, Cotte and Dupasquier (1916) reached the same conclusion on the basis of their experience. In Germany, a publication by Wederhake (1917) attracted much attention. He described favourable results obtained by grafting hernial sacs on skin defects. The hernial sac was obtained at operations for inguinal hernia. It was cut open and applied to the granulation tissue with the endothelial layer at the surface. According to Weder-

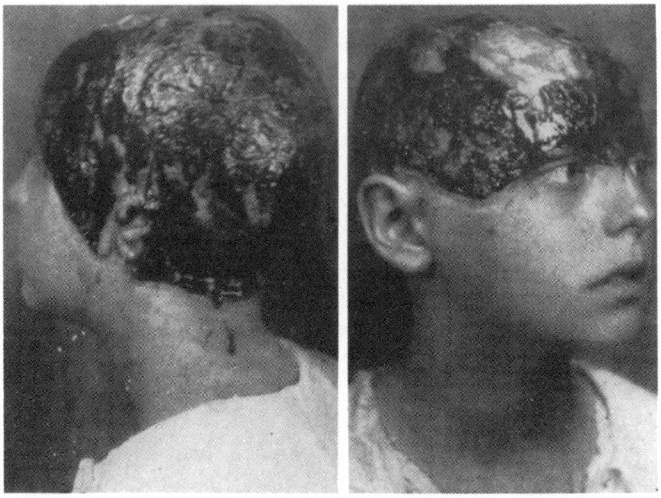

37 a

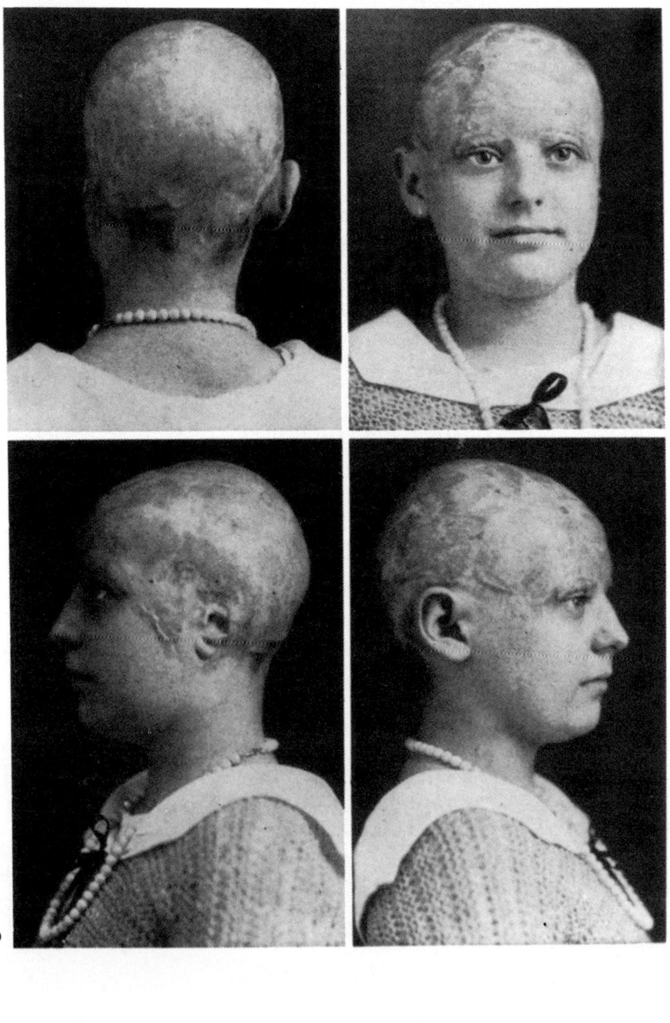

b

c
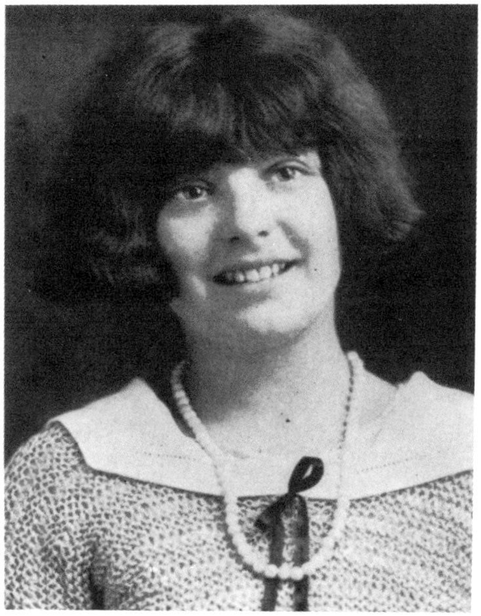

Fig. 37 a–c. Total avulsion of a girl's scalp with loss of the left ear and the eye brows. The skull is now covered with granulation tissue. Part of the skull lays bare because of avulsion of the pericranium **(a).** Healing was obtained in four months by six grafting procedures of which four autogenous partial thickness skin grafts were successful and two homografts failed **(b).** The same girl wearing a wig **(c)** (McWilliams 1924)

hake, the endothelium developed into epithelium. To ensure adequate adhesion between graft and wound, the latter was painted with serum. Grafts were applied also to suppurating wounds. After grafting, the "hernial sac graft" was painted with a tannin solution to harden the tissue. The value of a hernial sac as graft material was illustrated with five case histories of patients. Wederhake described the scars as being of good quality, and movable in relation to the underlying structure.

Lanz (1917), professor of surgery in Amsterdam, immediately responded to Wederhake's article. He stated that his teacher Kocher in Bern (Switzerland) had used hernial sac grafts as early as 1892. Lanz had been impressed at the time with the apparent metaplasia of endothelium to epithelium (which, on theoretical grounds, he understood to be impossible). To study this metaplasia, Lanz had examined biopsy specimens from the grafted area, and found progressive necrosis in all specimens. He reached the conclusion that "... der homöoplastisch transplantierte Bruchsack dient nur als Leitmembran, als Schrittmacher für das Epithelium; er bleibt als solcher sitzen." [14]

Subsequently, Lanz sometimes utilized this pacemaker property by covering large skin defects for which insufficient donor skin was available, with alternating strips of skin and hernial sac.

---

14 "The homogenously grafted hernial sac serves only as guide membrane, as pacemaker for the epithelium; as such it is accepted."

Lexer's assistant Keysser (1918) in Jena (Germany) also reacted to Wederhake's publication. He observed that, if Wederhake's contention was true, the rules formulated by Lexer would no longer apply. One of these rules was that only skin autografts could be successful. Keysser in any case criticized Wederhake's article severely because he (Wederhake) formulated a definite evaluation of the result within ten days of the operation. Keysser performed a more or less comparative study in order to establish whether serosa homografts were perhaps an exception to Lexer's rules. One of the patients he used for this purpose had burns, to which skin autografts and hernial sac homografts were applied simultaneously. Both graft types seemed to have taken seven days after the operation, but on the twelfth post-operative day the hernial sac detached itself. Bluish-white islands became visible in the granulation tissue beneath the hernial sac. Wederhake had misinterpreted these islands as epithelial islands. Biopsy specimens from this tissue showed that they consisted solely of young cicatricial tissue, without epithelium. Keysser concluded that serosa homografts did not differ from skin homografts. The organism reacted to hernial sac grafting with a foreign body reaction.

Views on Failures of Homografting

With the many disappointing results of homografting, views on the causes of failure gradually developed. Tinker and Prince (1911) had previously raised the question whether there were similarities between the processes which caused skin grafts to disappear and the haemolysis which occurred after some blood transfusions. The American Underwood of La Grande, Oregon, for example, attempted in 1914 to establish whether the clinical symptoms which developed in some patients after receiving several homografts might perhaps be due to anaphylactic reactions (Underwood 1914). [15] He had noticed that the clinical symptoms after repeated homografting seemed to show a close similarity to anaphylactic reactions. An investigation into possible similarities had never before been made.

Underwood described an example of a possible anaphylactic reaction in a patient with severe burns. This patient received the first homograft 12 days after the accident, and the procedure was subsequently repeated almost daily, with grafts obtained from relatives, friends and neighbours. Skin from 17 persons was thus grafted in 22 sessions. The grafts initially seemed to take well, but gradually all detached themselves. Underwood described this process as "melting away". The patient developed a number of conspicuous symptoms about three weeks after the first grafting. At sites at which epithelialization initially seemed to occur spontaneously, the granulation tissue became flaccid and started to bleed spontaneously. The patient developed haematuria and the body temperature rose to 39.4 °C while the heart action became quick and irregular. Leucocytopenia occurred, and the erythrocytes proved to contain purplish granules after staining. When these symptoms developed and the grafts disappeared for obscure reasons, Underwood dared not continue grafting. He assumed that the local and systemic reactions

15 The phenomenon of anaphylaxis attracted a lot of interest after the publication of Portier and Richet in 1902.

resulted from an anaphylactic reaction and wondered whether this reaction might be prevented by applying as much skin as possible in one session, or whether the patients could be desensitized.

Schlaepfer (1923) described a virtually identical syndrome after homografting. In his experience, homografts could suddenly become necrotic several months after the operation, and the patient in that case developed systemic toxic symptoms. He wondered whether there might be specific skin groups comparable with blood groups. Holman (1924) observed not only that homografting was virtually bound to fail but also that it could cause other complications. He himself described one of these complications. In a five-year-old girl with extensive skin defects resulting from an accident, the first homograft was applied 22 days after the accident, using skin from the mother, who had the same blood group as the child. The small deep grafts seemed to take, and more skin from the mother was grafted seven days later. All grafts again seemed to take, but three weeks after the first operation "exfoliative dermatitis" developed over the entire body surface, including the grafted area. The grafts and the epithelium which had formed around them disappeared. Spontaneous haemorrhages developed, and the faeces contained blood. The patient became febrile and had a rapid pulse.

Holman believed that the skin affection resulted from an anaphylactic reaction to foreign proteins. Three and a half months after the onset of dermatitis (the child was still ill), all remnants of the homografts were removed. The general condition improved within ten days and the skin lesions disappeared.

Holman concluded that the local and systemic symptoms could have been caused by intoxication or sensitization to foreign proteins. In his opinion, the patient could have been sensitized by the first homografting, while the second operation provoked the reaction. Holman considered it more plausible that the homografting had caused an immune reaction; in his opinion the degeneration of the grafts 10–12 days after the operation also pointed in this direction. Although the symptoms resembled an anaphylactic reaction, they were not identical to such a reaction. The immune reaction might express itself in systemic symptoms, but on the other hand might be confined to gradual disintegration of the grafts.

Keysser (1918) conducted several experiments to see whether the rejection of homografts might be prevented. In one of these experiments he transfused blood from the potential skin recipient to the potential skin donor. Prior to grafting, serum from the donor was applied to the wound surface to be grafted. Keysser gained the impression that the grafts then survived longer, but ultimately they did disintegrate.

On the basis of a study of the literature, Lehmann and Tammann (1926) had concluded that failure of skin homografting was due to an immunological reaction caused by the recipient. They were convinced that this immunological reaction was caused by the reticulo-endothelial system (RES) [16] and formulated the hypothesis that rejection of the skin homograft could be prevented by blockage of the RES. This hypothesis was tested in an experimental model. The RES in unrelated mice

16 The RES was described by Aschoff in 1924 and was experimented with to discover if a relationship existed between RES and homografting.

was blocked with trypan blue, and a skin homograft was performed. Although after acceptance the homografts behaved differently from autografts, part of the homografts remained vital according to their observations. The quality of the homografts, however, deteriorated in the course of three months.

Research into the value of RES blockage in homografting was continued by Tammann and Patrikelahis (1927). Instead of trypan blue, a colloidal solution of silver or copper was given by subcutaneous injection. In mice treated by RES blockage in this way, full-thickness skin grafts were likewise well accepted and seemed to remain vital. From the fifth week after grafting, the hair growth which had meanwhile resumed in the grafts became scantier, the skin adhered more firmly to the underlying structure and desquamation started. Microscopic examination 2–3 months after grafting showed that the subcutaneous adipose tissue had been replaced by densely cellularized connective tissue; the hair follicles had become atrophic, and the elastic fibres had hardly changed.

It was concluded from these two experiments that skin homografting in unrelated mice became possible when the RES was blocked. It was assumed that the changes which later occurred in the grafts resulted from diminished blocking of the RES.

Fischer (1929) continued the experiments, using rabbits and blocking the RES with benzol or benzene. He gained the impression that benzol/benzene inhibited the defense reaction, thus prolonging graft survival.

From Germany came other optimistic reports on the possibilities of homografting. Addressing the *Deutsche Gesellschaft für Chirurgie,* Mannheim (1930) maintained that he achieved permanent graft healing in patients treated by Braun's implantation method. In the course of the discussion of Mannheim's paper, only one member of the audience (Dzialoszynski 1930) remarked that permanent healing could never be expected after homografting, not even when the implantation method was used. A few years later, a publication from Lexer's department (Loeffler 1932) described the results of a similar experiment: the results of homografts performed by Braun's implantation method were proved not to differ from those of conventional homografts.

Study of the Histological Processes in Homografting

The histological processes involved in skin homografting were studied by several investigators, including Lexer's Japanese student Oshima (1914). He studied the behaviour of full-thickness skin grafts on a fresh wound bed. Marked degenerative changes were observed in the graft within nine days of grafting; the epidermis was much thinner than that of normal skin, and the nuclei of the epithelial cells showed marked atrophy. The sweat glands had already degenerated completely, and had been infiltrated by small cells. The connective tissue of the corium likewise already showed degenerative features: the fibres were swollen and the connective tissue cells stained poorly. Smooth muscle cells were no longer distinguishable after nine days. The blood vessels still contained vital erythrocytes, despite signs of endothelial degeneration.

After 16 days the nuclei of the epithelial cells could no longer be stained. Hair follicles were absent. Only vestiges of the sebaceous glands remained. In a biopsy specimen which Oshima obtained 28 days after grafting, epithelium was found to be entirely absent; the corium was infiltrated by cells; there were no blood vessels or glandular structures. The granulation tissue around the grafts contained numerous giant cells. Vestiges of connective tissue were still demonstrable 47 days after grafting.

Oshima (1914) concluded that the body responded to a homograft with a foreign body reaction. In his opinion the clinical features of a homograft did not reflect the situation found at histological examination.

The possibility of a foreign body reaction of the body in response to a homograft had been previously suggested by Papenhoff (1907), who also mentioned two further possibilities: a difference in blood composition between donor and recipient might give rise to a reaction which prevented permanent healing, or a difference in the protein composition of fluid between the homologous skin and the recipient might cause abnormal coagulation, permitting adhesion but not the establishment of circulatory continuity.

In 1916, Cotte and Dupasquier of Lyon studied the histological processes involved in homografting in a girl with a large defect of the hairy scalp resulting from an accident. Skin from a child deceased one hour after birth was applied to the granulating tissue. The grafts seemed to take well but, about 15 days after the operation, seemed to disappear as a result of absorption. Small ulcers formed at the graft edges. Biopsy specimens were taken from these ulcers for histological examination. The absorption was found to be caused by a considerable number of macrophages which had broken down the epithelial barrier, dislocated the basilar bed and invaded the skin tissue, thus hastening elimination of the last vestiges of the graft. The existence of young connective tissue with scattered fibroblasts in some points showed the onset of repair.

Subsequently, another attempt was made with skin from a 10-year-old child. This skin was first frozen for three days. Seven days later the graft had taken, but symptoms of absorption developed 16 days later. The epidermis of the graft disappeared, and the remainder assumed a blue colour. At microscopic examination, "no vestiges of cutaneous elements were found, the whole space being filled with young connective tissue originating in the granular bed". Cotte and Dupasquier concluded that homografts initially seemed to take but then disintegrated by an unknown process and were absorbed by leucocytes.

Holman (1924) undoubtedly made the most unequivocal statement about the possibilities of homografting: "... successful isografts (=homografts) exist only in fable and not in fact."

References

Alglave P (1907) Réparation des pertes de substance cutanée par des semis dermo-épidermiques suivant un procédé dérivé de celui de Jacques Reverdin. Bull Soc Anat Paris 82:251–255

Alglave P (1917) De la Réparation des substances cutanées par des semis dermo-épidermiques. Presse Med 25:419

Archer CW (1917) Skingrafting. Lancet 2:133

Bettman AG (1927) A new Thiersch graft razor. JAMA 89:451

Bier A (1918) Beobachtungen über Regeneration beim Menschen. Dtsch Med Wochenschr 44:1209

Blair VP (1924 a) Full thickness skin graft. Ann Surg 80:298–324

Blair VP (1924 b) The influence of mechanical pressure on wound healing. Ill Med J 45: 249–252

Blair VP, Brown JB (1929) The use and uses of large split-skin grafts of intermediate thickness. Surg Gynecol Obstet 49:82–97

Braun W (1920) Zur Technik der Hautpfropfung. Zentralbl Chir 47:1555

Calot F (1913) Une nouvelle méthode de greffes dermo-épidermiques. Belg Med 20:19

Carrel A (1912) The preservation of tissues and its application in surgery. JAMA 59:523–527

Cassegrain OC (1924) The small deep graft experience and results of the last three years. Surg Gynecol Obstet 38:557–559

Chaussy (1907) Ueber Krauselappen bei Ulcus cruris. Muench Med Wochenschr 54:1980

Coller FA (1925) The use of paraffin as a primary dressing for skin grafts. Surg Gynecol Obstet 41:221–225

Conynham EF (1913) Safety-razor to cut Thiersch grafts. JAMA 60:1245

Cotte G, Dupasquier (1916) A propos de deux tentatives de greffes cutanées homoplastiques: étude histologique. Lyon Chir 13:947–956

Cullen TS (1924) A progressively enlarging ulcer of the abdominal wall involving the skin and fat, following drainage of an abdominal abscess apparently of appendiceal origin. Surg Gynecol Obstet 38:579–582

Davis JS (1909 a) A method of splinting skin graft. Ann Surg 49:416–418

Davis JS (1909 b) The effect of scarlet red in various combinations, upon the epitheliation of granulating surfaces. Bull Johns Hopkins Hosp 20:176–180

Davis JS (1910) A method of splinting skin grafts. Bull Johns Hopkins Hosp 15:44

Davis JS (1911) Scalping accidents. Bull Johns Hopkins Hosp 16:257–362

Davis JS (1912) Discussion: the preservation of tissues and its application in surgery. (Carrel) JAMA 59:523

Davis JS (1914) The use of small deep skin grafts. JAMA 63:985–989

Davis JS (1917) The use of free grafts of whole thickness skin for the relief of contractures. Surg Gynecol Obstet 25:1

Davis JS (1919) Plastic surgery; its principles and practise. Kimpton, London

Davis JS (1929) The small deep graft: relationship to Reverdin graft. Ann Surg 89:902–916

Davis JS, Traut HF (1925) Origin and development of the blood supply of whole-thickness skin grafts. Ann Surg 82:871–879

Davis JS, Traut HF (1926) A method of obtaining greater relaxation with whole thickness skin grafts. Surg Gynecol Obstet 42:710

Dehelly G (1922) La greffe cutanée de Davis. Bull Soc Chir Paris 48:495–502

Douglas B (1923) Skin grafting by exact pattern. Ann Surg 77:223–227

Douglas B (1930) The sieve-graft – a stable transplant for covering large skin defects. Surg Gynecol Obstet 50:1018–1023

Douglas SR, Colebrook L, Fleming A (1917) On skin-grafting: a plea for its more extensive application. Lancet 2:5–12

Dowd CN (1906) The use of Wolfe grafts and tendon-lengthening in treating cicatricial contractures. Ann Surg 43:278–287

Dubreuilh W, Noël P (1911) Greffe cutanée par transplantation totale ou lambeau non pédiculé. Rev Chir (Paris) 43:82–113

Dubreuilh W (1919) Greffes de Reverdin par un procédé nouveau. J Med Bordeaux Sud-Ouest 50:545

Dzanelidze YY (1952) Swobodnaya peresadka kozie. (Free skin grafting) in Russian. Medhiez (Medical State Publishing Company), Moscow

Dzialoszynski A (1930) Discussion: Homoïoplastische und heteroplastische Hauttransplantation beim Menschen (Mannheim). Langenbecks Arch Chir 162:151

Enderlen D (1912) Methodik und praktische Bedeutung der Transplantation. Z Aertzl Fortbild 9:737–744

Esser JFS (1916) Neue Wege für Chirurgische Plastiken durch Heranziehung der Zahnärztliche Technik. Bruns' Beitr Klin Chir 103:547–555
Esser JFS (1917 a) Studies in plastic surgery of the face. Ann Surg 65:297–315
Esser JFS (1917 b) Sogenannte totale Ösophagusplastik aus Hautlappen nach Thiersch ohne Verwendung von Darmschlinge. Dtsch Z Chir 142:403–410
Esser JFS (1917 c) Urinblasenersatz bei Ectopia vesicae. Zentralbl Chir 44:937
Esser JFS (1922) Einfache Rettung aus schwieriger Lage bei Gesichtsverstümmelung durch „Epitheleinlage". Zentralbl Chir 49:1217–1219
Finochietto E (1922) Rasoir avec dispositif pour tailler des greffes d'une épaisseur regulière. Bull Soc Chir Paris 48:450
Fischer H (1929) Tierexperimentelle Studien zum Problem der Homoïotransplantation. Langenbecks Arch Chir 156:224–250
Flick K (1930) Verfahren zur Entnahme grosser Epidermislappen. Dtsch Z Chir 222:302–305
Föderl O (1905) Messer zur Bildung Thierschscher Transplantationslappen. Wien Klin Wochenschr 25:677
Gatch WD (1911) Report of a case of extensive Tiersch skin graft. Bull Johns Hopkins Hosp 22:84
Gillies HD (1918) Discussions on plastic operations of the eyelids. Trans Ophthalmol Soc UK 38:70–99
Gillies HD (1920) Plastic surgery of facial burns. Surg Gynecol Obstet 30:121
Gillies HD, Kilner TP (1929) Symblepharon; its treatment by Thiersch and mucous membrane grafting. Trans Ophthalmol Soc UK 49:470–479
Gluck T (1906) Transplantation der Haut von einer Leiche. Zentralbl Chir 33:679
Gould EP, Archer CW (1915) Local anaesthesia in skin-grafting by Thiersch's method. Br Med J 1:544
Greenfield DG (1917) A note on skin grafting. Br Med J 1:482
Haberer H (1904) Einige Fälle ausgedehnter Hauttransplantation nach Thiersch. Dtsch Med Wochenschr 30:551–555
Hagen GL (1924) Dermotome. JAMA 82:1933
Halsted WS (1913) Development in the skin-grafting operation for cancer of the breast. JAMA 60:416–418
Hofmann M (1907) Gedecktes Transplantationsmesser. Zentralbl Chir 34:318
Holman E (1924) Protein sensitization in isoskingrafting. Surg Gynecol Obstet 38:100–106
Holman E (1925) Restoration of the scalp. JAMA 84:350–352
Holzapfel (1916) Mehr Transplantieren. Muench Med Wochenschr 63:1469
Iselin H (1916) Transplantation freier Hautlappen zwecks oberflächlicher Fettaufpflanzung. Brun's Beitr Klin Chir 102:721
Joseph J (1918) Ungewöhnlich grosse Gesichtsplastik. Dtsch Med Wochenschr 44:465
Joynt RL (1928) A new method of cutting large skin grafts. Lancet 1:816
Keysser Fr (1918) Bewertung neuerer chirurgischer Transplantationsbestrebungen. Bruns' Beitr Klin Chir 110:660–671
Kilner TP, Jackson T (1921) Skin-grafting in buccal cavity. Br J Surg 9:148–154
Koch SL (1926) The covering of raw surfaces with particular reference to the hand. Surg Gynecol Obstet 43:677–686
Krause F (1893) Ueber die Transplantation grosser ungestielter Hautlappen. Verh Dtsch Ges Chir 22:46
Kubányi A (1924) Hauttransplantationsversuche auf Grundlage der Isoagglutination. Langenbecks Arch Chir 129:644–647
Lanz O (1907) Over transplantatie. (On skin grafting) in Dutch. Ned Tijdschr Geneesk 51:1335–1337
Lanz O (1908) Die Transplantation betreffend. Zentralbl Chir 35:3
Lanz O (1917) Der Bruchsack im Dienste der Transplantation. Zentralbl Chir 44:761
Lauenstein C (1912) Zur Frage der Überpflanzung behaarter Haut. Zentralbl Chir 39:1220
Law AA (1915) The clinical status of the autograft. Ann Surg 62:602–609
Lehmann W, Tammann H (1925) Transplantation und Vitalspeicherung. Bruns' Beitr Klin Chir 135:259–302
Lexer E (1919) Die freien Transplantationen, part 1. Enke, Stuttgart

Lexer E (1925) 20 Jahre Transplantationsforschung in der Chirurgie. Langenbecks Arch Chir 138:251–302
Loeb L (1930) Transplantation and individuality. Physiol Rev 10:547–616
Loeffler (1932) Die Auto- und homoplastische Epidermisimplantation. Dtsch Z Chir 236:169–190
Mannheim H (1930) Homoïplastische und heteroplastische Hauttransplantation beim Menschen. Langenbecks Arch Chir 162:551–560
de Martigny F (1913) De la transplantation homogène de peau conservée en chambre froide. Cong Franç Chir 26:252–255
Masson JC (1918) Skin grafting. JAMA 70:1581–1584
McWilliams CA (1924) Principles of the four types of skin grafting. JAMA 83:183–189
McWilliams CA (1926) Free, full-thickness skin grafts. Ann Surg 84:237–245
Meyer H (1930) Discussion: Homoïplastische und heteroplastische Hauttransplantation beim Menschen (Mannheim). Langenbecks Arch Chir 162:149
Moss WL (1917) Simplified method for determining the iso-agglutinin group in the selection of donors for blood transfusion. JAMA 68:1905
Moszkowicz L (1917) Ueber Verpflanzung Thiersch'scher Epidermis Läppchen in die Mundhöhle. Langenbecks Arch Chir 108:216
Müller A (1912) Ueber die Deckung von Harnröhrendefekten mittels Thierscher Transplantation. Dtsch Med Wochenschr 38:2307
Nicoladoni C (1900) Daumenplastik und organischer Ersatz der Fingerspitze (Anticheiroplastik und Daktyloplastik). Langenbecks Arch Chir 61:606
Obituary (1928) R. L. Joynt. Lancet 1:836
Oshima T (1914) Ueber das Schicksal des homoïoplastisch transplantierten Hautlappens beim Menschen. Langenbecks Arch Chir 103:440–470
Papenhoff H (1907) Ueber Transplantation eigener und fremder Haut und die Ursachen für die Nichtanheilung der letzteren. Inaugural thesis, Albert-Ludwigs Universität Freiburg, Rebholtz, Freiburg in Breisgau
Parce AD (1922) An improved method of skin-grafting. Ann Surg 75:658–662
Perimoff V (1913) Zur Frage der Überpflanzung behaarter Haut. Zentralbl Chir 40:1443
Perthes G (1917) Ist homöoplastische Hautverpflanzung unter Geschwistern der Autotransplantation gleichwertig? Zentralbl Chir 44:426
Reid MR (1922) The use of large Reverdin grafts in the healing of chronic osteomyelitis. Bull Johns Hopkins Hosp 33:386–388
Reschke K (1922) Injektions Epithelisierung nach Pels-Leusden. Ein neues Verfahren, granulierende Flächen und Wunden zu überhäuten. Bruns' Beitr Klin Chir 127:647–656
Rulison ET (1927) The postoperative care of Ollier-Thiersch skin grafts; advisability of daily surgical dressings. Surg Gynecol Obstet 45:708–710
Sabella N (1913) Use of the fetal membranes in skin grafting. Med Rec (1866–1922) 83: 478–480
Schepelmann E (1911) Über Thierschsche Hautverpflanzung. Med Klin (Munich) 7:1048
Schlaepfer K (1923) Closure of granulating wounds with Reverdin-Halsted grafts. Bull Johns Hopkins Hosp 34:114–118
Schöne G (1912) Die heteroplastische und homöoplastische Transplantation. Springer, Berlin
Schöne G (1915) Ueber Tiefenwachstum des Epithels nach Thiersch verpflanzter Epidermisläppchen. Bruns' Beitr Klin Chir 95:317–323
Shawan HK (1919) The principle of blood grouping applied to skingrafting. JAMA 157: 503–509
Smith F (1926 a) A rational management of skin grafts. Surg Gynecol Obstet 42:556–562
Smith F (1926 b) Pressure bags for skin grafting. Surg Gynecol Obstet 43:99
Smythe FW (1922) Simple protection for newly placed skin grafts. JAMA 78:1963
Sneve H (1905) The treatment of burns and skingrafting. JAMA 45:1–8
Sokolof NW (1925) Die Bedeutung der organspezifischen Immunität und biochemischen Struktur des Blutes für die Homotransplantation. Z Immunitatesforsch 42:44
Sonnenburg E, Tschmarke P (1915) Die Verbrennungen und Erfrierungen. Enke, Stuttgart
Stern M (1913) The grafting of preserved amniotic membrane to burned and ulcerated surfaces substituting skin grafts. JAMA 60:973

Tammann H, Patrikalakis M (1927) Weitere Versuche über homoïoplastische Hauttransplantationen bei Vitalspeicherung. Bruns' Beitr Klin Chir 139:550–568
Tinker MB, Prince HL (1911) Modified autogenous and turning skinflaps to cover granulating surfaces. Ann Surg 54:848–853
Torrance G (1920) Skin grafting by means of freezing with ethyl chloride. Surg Gynecol Obstet 30:405
Underwood HL (1914) Anaphylaxis following skin-grafting for burns. JAMA 63:775
de Waard (1930) De epitheliumplastiek van Braun. (Transplantation of epithelium by Braun method) in Dutch. Geneesk Tijdschr Ned-Indie 70:1050
Wangensteen OH (1930) The implantation method of skin grafting. Surg Gynecol Obstet 50: 634–638
Wederhake (1917) Die Anwendung von Bruchsäcken zur Transplantation. Muench Med Wochenschr 64:785–788
Wehle F (1922) A successful skingraft with a slight modification of the Reverdin method. Med Rec (1866–1922) 101:587
Wiener J (1913) Skin-grafting without dressings. JAMA 60:1526
Willis AM (1925) The value of debridement in the treatment of burns. JAMA 84:655–658
Wydler A (1914) Über den Schutz der Thiersch'schen Transplantation mit Korkpapier. Zentralbl Chir 41:3–5

Chapter 6
Skin Grafting During the Period 1930–1950

Differentiation of the indications for and the applications of skin grafts took place during the period 1930–1950. Several factors played a role in this evolution: improved technique, specialization by some surgeons, and improved preoperative, peroperative and postoperative care. The number of patients requiring operative treatment of skin defects increased, partly also as a result of the events of World War II; the experience gained by surgeons who had to treat these injuries increased proportionally.

A. Split-Skin Grafts

Indications

Burns continued to be the most common indication for skin grafting. Early excision, as already outlined by Willis in 1925 (see Chap. 5) was not yet accepted routine as would appear from the publication by Brown and McDowell of St. Louis, Missouri, in 1942. Grafting was usually done after granulation tissue had developed. According to Allen and Koch (1942) of Chicago (Illinois) this situation was generally reached after 20–35 days. The grafts were applied to the granulation tissue, although these grafts were known to give far from perfect results. The chance of acceptance was nearly 100%, and the main objective was to close the defects as quickly as possible.

This principle was not infrequently abandoned when facial burns were involved; thick split-skin grafts were used for these injuries by Padgett (1942) of Kansas City, Missouri.

When the burns had healed by second intention or when thin grafts had been used to close the defects, reconstructive surgery was required later when the integument was insufficient, contractures developed or the appearance was unsatisfactory. Padgett advocated the use of three-quarter-thickness skin grafts for reconstruction in these cases. He also used grafts of this type in the face, e.g. in ectropion of the eyelids. Although these grafts hardly contracted, a second operation was not infrequently necessary when a hypertrophic scar had formed.

Carcinomatous degeneration (epidermoid or basal cell carcinoma) in old unhealed burns was treated by ample excision, whereupon the defects were closed with grafts (Browne 1941).

Skin lesions caused by radium or roentgen rays were sometimes also regarded as burns. Most patients in this category had been exposed to soft rays in the days when X-rays were still rather negligently used. Gillies and McIndoe[1] (1935) divided these patients into three groups:

a) Those exposed to a single diagnostic or therapeutic dose
b) Those exposed to frequent small doses for treatment of a chronic condition (usually resulting in ulcers)
c) Those who had handled X-rays professionally.

Indications for operative treatment were: pain, pruritus, ulceration, deformity from contracture, cosmetic appearance and epitheliomatous changes (Braun 1934; Gillies and McIndoe 1935; Padgett 1942). After excision of the affected tissue, the defects were covered with split-skin grafts or with flaps.

As during the period 1900–1930, much attention was focused also on the use of skin grafts to reline cavities such as eye sockets and gingivo-labial sulci. Padgett initially used three-quarter-thickness skin grafts for this purpose, but later he switched to thin grafts (Padgett 1942, 1946) and joined his contemporaries (McIndoe 1937; Kilner 1948), who followed the advice of a pioneer in this field (Esser 1916). For cavity grafting, the advice was to make a larger cavity than was actually required. This over-distension had to be maintained for some considerable time (6 weeks to 4 months), lest the cavity become too small as a result of contraction (McIndoe 1937). McIndoe (1937) and Matthews (1943) used this method in, for example, the treatment of destruction of the buccal sulcus by tuberculosis. The graft was not affected by tuberculous inflammation. Elderly persons whose teeth had been extracted and whose buccal sulcus became too shallow for the proper fitting of dentures, were greatly helped by deepening the sulcus with the aid of grafts. Also, retrognathia could be simply corrected with the aid of a large buccal inlay, with fair results. McIndoe considered it possible to use an epithelial inlay for reconstruction of hypospadias, particularly in men who had already undergone several unsuccessful operations in childhood, and in whom a flap had likewise failed to produce a fair result. He used a closed method with the aid of an "introducer" on which a graft was mounted. The canal for a new urethra was made with the introducer (which resembled a trocar). A catheter was left in situ for 3–4 months in the newly formed urethra in order to prevent contraction of the grafts. The epithelial inlay was also employed in the construction of an artificial vagina in cases of atresia (McIndoe and Banister 1938).

A paper which Kilner (1948) read at a meeting of the Ophthalmological Society of the United Kingdom shows that the treatment of the contracted eyesocket still constituted a problem; particularly in patients who had lost an eye in the war of 1914–1918. The size of the eyesocket in these patients had diminished. The relining was done with the aid of thin skin grafts, and the conjunctival deficiency was, if

1 The names of Gillies, Kilner and McIndoe will be mentioned several times in this section. All three played an important role in the development of plastic surgery. Sidcup (where Gillies and Kilner worked) and East Grinstead (where McIndoe worked) became renowned not only in Britain but throughout the whole world.

necessary, similarly treated with the aid of grafts. The mould used in these operations was flask-shaped and had been evolved by Ascott.

Ulcers of the lower leg of course continued to give the surgeons concern. It was agreed that the underlying condition was of little importance for treatment. Regardless of whether the ulcer had formed on the basis of mechanical damage, common or specific inflammatory processes or venous insufficiency, excision and grafting remained the treatment of choice. For venous ulcers the advice was to improve the venous situation by ligating the great saphenous vein or sclerosing the dilatated veins.

Apart from a whole range of other applications already mentioned in preceding chapters, grafts were used to close skin defects resulting from excision of birthmarks, tumours (e.g. mammary tumours, Goode 1935) and redundant tissue in rhinophyma (Padgett 1942).

Grafting Technique

General Measures Prior to Skin Grafting

Ever since before World War II, the possibilities of improving the patient's condition for the operation received more attention. It was known from experience that patients weakened by long suffering tended to develop infections. Anaemia was regarded as a contra-indication to operative treatment (Ludwig 1946).

According to Padgett (1942), the risk of infection increased by a factor of 2 or 3 when the haemoglobin concentration was less than 65%. Hypoproteinaemia (Cannon et al. 1944) and dehydration were also considered to be unfavourable factors. Moreover, an optimal diet with sufficient vitamins, fluids and electrolytes was advocated (Padgett 1942).

Preparation of the Grafted Area

Clean traumatic wounds or fresh surgical wounds were preferably covered with grafts as soon as adequate haemostasis was achieved. If no adequate haemostasis could be achieved or if the wound floor was of poor quality, e.g. after operations in cicatricial tissue, grafting was sometimes postponed a few days. Infected wounds were not covered with grafts as long as clinical evidence of infection was present. Infected necrotic tissue was excised, and an expectant attitude was taken until granulation tissue of "good" quality had developed (Padgett 1937, 1942).

It generally took 2–3 weeks to bring an infection under control. The appearance of the wound was considered more important than the outcome of bacterial cultures (Padgett 1942; Buff 1952). The desired condition of the granulation tissue was brought about with the aid of dressings moistened every hour with an antiseptic solution, e.g. Dakin's, azochloramide, hexylmethylamine or saturated boric acid solution (Conway and Coldwater 1946). When the appearance of the wound improved too slowly, heat was also applied. Wounds which showed hypergranulation were treated with pressure bandages.

After World War II new antiseptics such as acriflavine and quatenary ammonium compounds were developed, by which disinfection was facilitated.

Anaesthesia

The operations were performed under general as well as under local anaesthesia, but the search for other, simpler techniques of anaesthesia continued. One of the lines of research concerned the practical use of the anaesthetic properties of cold (Mock 1943). It was found that, if the donor site was covered with icepacks (under some pressure, if possible) two hours before the grafts were cut, anesthesia for about 20 minutes was achieved. In this way, Mock achieved complete anaesthesia in 24 of the 27 donor sites so prepared.

Instruments

The need for good instruments greatly increased as the range of indications for skin grafting widened and the number of surgeons performing skin grafts increased. The cutting of grafts also requires skill.

Several proposals for improvement of graft-cutting instruments had already been made during the first decades of the 20th century but nevertheless the razor continued to be the instrument most widely used for this purpose. Developments continued during and after the thirties. Humby (1934) of Guy's Hospital (see Fig. 38) formulated several criteria for graft-cutting instruments. His first and most important criterion was error-proof use. It had to be possible to cut large grafts with the instrument from curving surfaces, e.g. the thigh, for instance by flattening this surface. Displacement of the skin in relation to underlying structures had to be prevented during cutting. This meant that the donor site had to be fixed, but not so

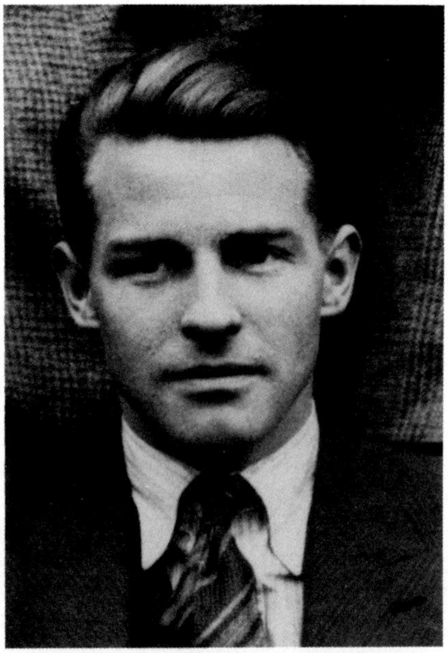

Fig. 38. Graham Humby, designer of the skin grafting knife while he was a medical student at Guy's Hospital

forcibly as to damage it. The grafts had to be of uniform thickness and width. The knife had to remain sharp, and sterilization of the dermatome had to be simple. On the basis of these criteria Humby designed a voluminous apparatus (Fig. 39 a + b) which consisted of a framework that could be taped to the extremity. Crossbars at the ends of the frame carried small needles, which could be pushed down into the skin and stretched the skin when the frame was extended. A disposable knife could slide in the framework. The angle between knife and cut surface was adjustable, and a rollerbar was mounted 0.3 cm in front of the knife.

This instrument evidently was not too satisfactory, for in 1936 Humby introduced a greatly simplified modified version of the original instrument (Fig. 39 c). This modified version became known as the "Humby knife" and consisted of a blade with grip. A roller-bar was mounted in front of the blade, and cutting depth could be adjusted with the aid of screws on the roller-bar. The knife had to be sharpened with a whetstone.

One of the major complaints of users of graft-cutting instruments was that the knives tended to be dull. Several suggestions were therefore made to use disposable blades (Müller Meernach 1942; Brown and McDowell 1943; Webster 1945; Bodenham 1949). The blade proposed by the German Müller Meernach was nothing but a cheap wooden potato-peeler in which one half of a safety-razor blade fitted; it cost 9 pfennigs. In Brown and McDowell's monograph, *Skingrafting of burns* (1943), an illustration showed the skin-grafting instrument designed by Ferris Smith; it consisted of a ribbed back and a straight-razor blade with a length of 18 cm, which could be exchanged. Apart from proposals for disposable blades, efforts were made to improve their cutting depth. This was usually attempted by fitting a roller-bar in front of the blade and a mechanism by which the distance between blade and roller-bar could be adjusted (Marcks 1943). The instrument designed by Lagrot (1947) also had a mechanism for adjustment of cutting depth, but neither his description nor that published by Dufourmentel (1950) makes it clear whether the blade could be exchanged. Several aids were used to flatten the donor area during graft cutting, e.g. an assistant's hand, a wooden board, a special serrated device (Kilner and Jackson 1921) or a suction box. Gabarro (1944) devised a still widely used steel board with four different notches which, when pushed down, flattened a skin surface area as wide as the notch. Much earlier, Flick (1930) had proposed the subcutaneous insertion of a Kirschner wire cranial and caudal to the donor site. The donor area was stretched flat by pulling on braces fitted to the ends of the Kirschner wire.

The method was again recommended almost 20 years later by Clery in 1949.

In 1947 Barker designed a dermatome which combined a blade with a suction cup, and which he called a "vacuotome" (Barker 1948 b, 1950). The cutting depth was adjustable and the vacuotome was as used by several surgeons, including some Europeans (Schuchardt 1949).

The American Padgett (Fig. 40) was among the surgeons who had great difficulties in cutting grafts of uniform thickness and reasonable dimensions. Like many others, therefore, he was looking for a dermatome which would minimize the risk of technical errors. He discussed his wishes with Professor Hood, mechanical engineer, who like himself was working at the University of Kansas. From 1930 on they made efforts to design a dermatome which was simple to operate and could

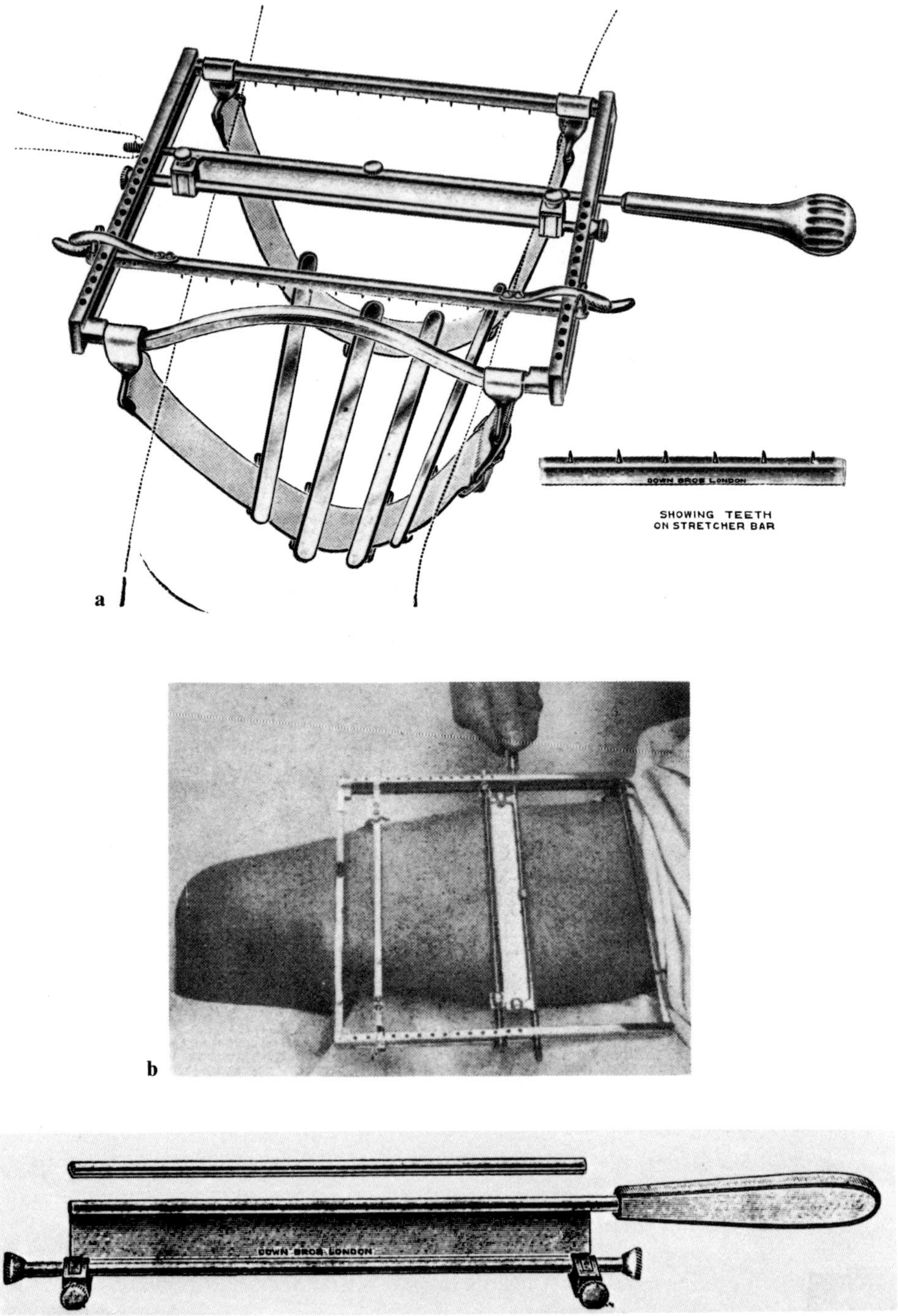

Fig. 39 a – c. Humby's first design for a dermatome. **a** an illustration from a commercial catalogue, **b** dermatome fixed to a leg with slings, ready for use (Humby 1934). The simplified model of the Humby knife (Humby 1936)

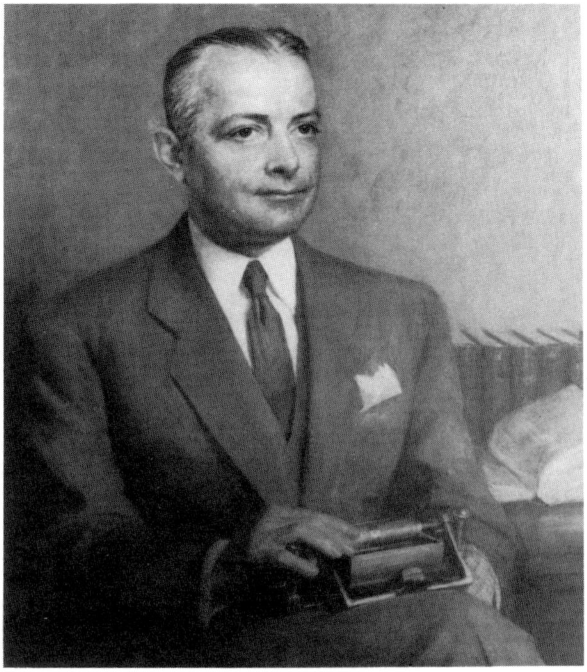

Fig. 40. Earl Calvin Padgett (1893 – 1946). In this portrait together with the dermatome which he developed

cut grafts of a uniform, readily adjustable thickness. It was not until 1938 that a useful result was obtained.

Unlike all the other dermatomes designed at that time, this consisted of a semicircular drum and a blade (Fig. 41). The distance between drum and blade was adjustable. In principle, the grafts cut were the same size as the drum. The skin to be cut was cemented onto the drum, and this made it superfluous to stretch the skin; grafts could therefore be cut from virtually any site. The device also made it possible to cut grafts of a particular shape. The skin to be left in situ was painted with talcum and ether, and consequently did not adhere to the drum (and was not cut off). Grafts of any desired thickness could be cut with this dermatome. Padgett (1942, 1946) himself distinguished four graft types which could be cut with his dermatome:

1) Thiersch grafts with a thickness of 0.2–0.25 mm
2) Superficial and intermediate split-skin grafts which were 0.3–0.4 mm thick and comprised one-third to two-thirds of the entire skin thickness
3) Three-quarter-thickness skin grafts which were 0.5–0.6 mm thick and comprised 75%–90% of the skin thickness
4) Full-thickness skin grafts which were 0.88–1 mm thick.

In selecting graft thickness, Padgett took several factors into account, including the quality of the wound floor. For fresh wounds which required a graft that caused only slight contraction and ensured a good cosmetic result, he selected grafts with a

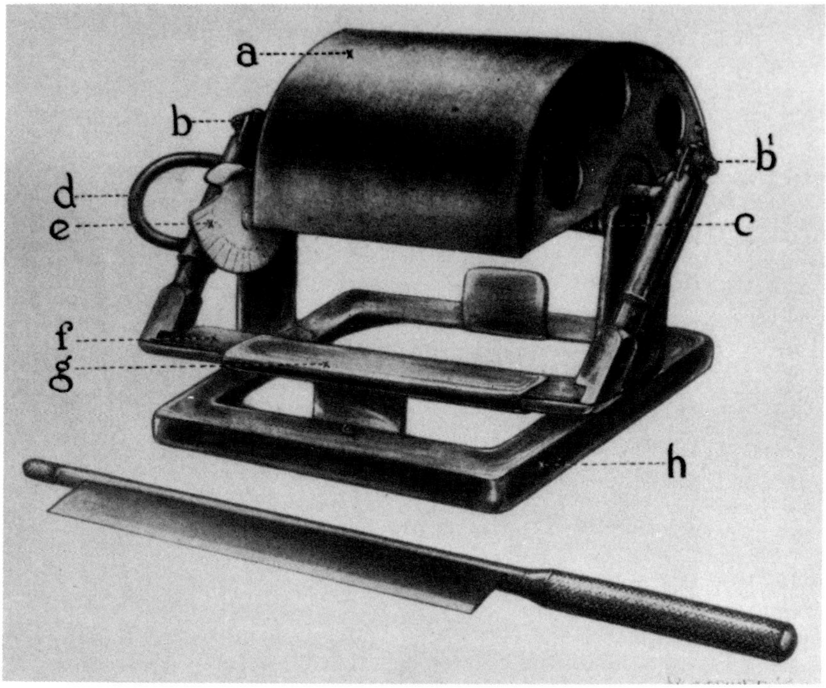

Fig. 41. One of the early versions of the Padgett-Hood dermatome (Padgett 1942)

thickness of 0.5–0.6 mm. For sites at which contraction (if any) would cause no serious complications, he used grafts of 0.41–0.50 mm thickness in the treatment of women and children. Padgett's grafting results improved substantially after the introduction of this dermatome, particularly in patients with clean, fresh wounds, to which three-quarter-thickness skin grafts were applied.

Padgett's precise definition of the various skin graft thicknesses was considered impracticable by many surgeons, who thought that so highly differentiated a method of cutting was not feasible. They pointed out that, for example, the thickness of the cement layer on the drum influenced the thickness of the graft to be cut (Converse and Robb-Smith 1944; Robinson 1949). Brown and McDowell (1943) and Barker (1948 b) advised that the blade always be kept as close to the drum as possible, because the dermatome always cut too deep. The attempts made by Brown and McDowell (1943) to calibrate the grafts failed because in their opinion the skin thickness varied too much with the patient's race, age and nutritional condition. They therefore distinguished only between split-thickness skin grafts and full-thickness skin grafts. Their split-thickness skin grafts included Ollier-Thiersch grafts, razor grafts, epidermic garfts, blanket grafts and implantation grafts, and generally comprised some 80% of the corium.

Padgett and Hood's principle of skin fixation for graft cutting had already been described in various other ways, e.g. by Eymer. Eymer had also proceeded from the postulate that a graft of uniform thickness could only be cut if the skin was completely fixed in relation to the blade. In his dermatome (Fig. 42), a metal plate flattened the skin, and the blade – mounted on the plate via a guide-roller – cut through the skin at a fixed distance immediately beneath and parallel to the plate. Eymer's dermatome received hardly any attention, probably because its use was too difficult.

Padgett's dermatome still had some disadvantages, and modifications were soon suggested. One of the objections made concerned the fact that the blade could not be exchanged. The blade dulled quickly and it was difficult to sharpen it. The obvious solution seemed to be to replace the fixed blade by a blade carrier with disposable blades (Shumacker 1944; Marino 1948; Barker 1948 c). The Argentinian Marino (1948) had discussed the blade problem in correspondence with Padgett, and from this correspondence we know why Padgett himself did not introduce this modification. On 13th July 1943 Padgett wrote to Marino: "We have never been able to get a satisfactory blade. The reason for this is that just about the time we started getting the dermatome into production, the war came on and because of the high priorities required on steel the various steel companies did not want to fool with extra nick-nacks." Marino found the Argentinian steel industry willing to produce the desired disposable blades.

Another addition to the dermatome was a mirror mounted on the cutting arm, which gave the surgeon a better view of the field of operation (Jenney 1945; Aufricht and Dowd 1948). Robinson (1948) proposed various modifications which Hood carried out (Padgett died in 1946). Hood replaced the copper drum by one of aluminium; cement adhered better to aluminium, and the dermatome became less heavy. He also replaced the adjustable screws on either side of the drum by an adjusting mechanism on one side.

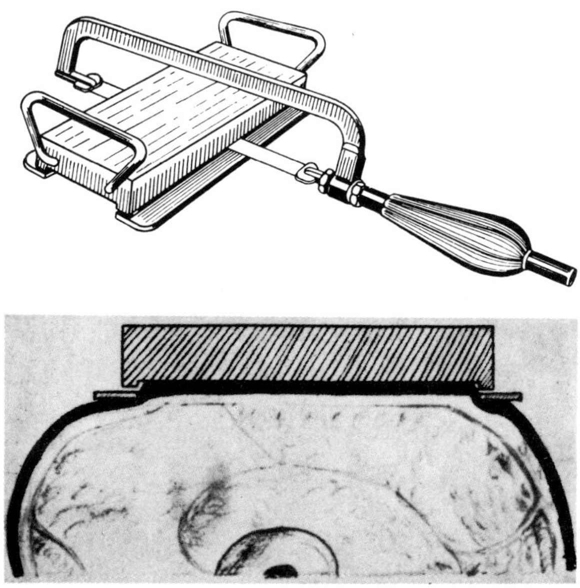

Fig. 42. Eymer's dermatome; the skin was flattened by a metal plate, from under which the graft was cut (Eymer 1935)

Apart from the technical modifications, several variants of the Padgett dermatome were designed, e.g. by Marino (1948), who introduced the so-called half-size dermatome, which was particularly suitable for use on children. The counterpart of this small dermatome was the giant dermatome which Hood designed (Litton and Hood 1954). In this giant dermatome, the semicircular drum was replaced by a cylinder. Large grafts could be cut with it, and this did away with one of the objections made to the Padgett dermatome: that only relatively small grafts could be cut with it (Schuchardt 1949). The giant dermatome however could only be used on a few areas. An original suggestion to enhance the graft yield with a Padgett dermatome had been made by Zintel (1945). He wondered whether a graft still adhering to the drum, could be split by cutting it once more, with the blade adjusted more economically; this would produce a graft twice as large, which he called split split-thickness skin graft.

One of the gravest problems in the use of the Padgett dermatome was how to loosen the graft from the drum without tearing it. This inconvenience could be overcome by applying to the drum, prior to cutting, a material which could later be removed along with the graft (Webster 1944 b; Jenney 1945; Reese 1946; Singer 1954). Materials used for this purpose were pliofilm or cellophane (Webster) and fine cotton bobbinet (Jenney). Reese found pliofilm too thin and too vulnerable, and advocated dermatape – a single-layer specially woven material. Berkow (1945) designed a special dermatome following the same principle in order to ensure optimal use of the tape on the grafts.

Also in the forties, Brown evolved the electrical dermatome (Brown 1948; Meloy and Letterman 1950). It was recommended as a "surprisingly safe instrument in the hands of the novice". For the more experienced surgeon, it was considered suitable for cutting grafts in infants and small children. Several other electrical dermatomes were subsequently devised (e.g. by Gosset 1952), which made it possible to adjust not only the thickness but also the width of the grafts.

Selection of Donor Sites

After the introduction of the Padgett dermatome, donor sites other than the conventional sites, e.g. the thigh, were more intensively used. It has already been pointed out that this was possible mainly because the skin no longer had to be stretched. Padgett preferred the abdominal wall. Others preferred the skin of the back, where both the corium and the epidermis were thick. Moreover, epithelialization occurred quickly after graft cutting, and consequently this donor site could be used several times. In some cases the same donor site was used five times in succession, always with an interval of 19 days (Brown and McDowell 1942 b, 1943).

Grateful use was made of Barker's suggestion (1948 a) to flatten the donor site in emaciated persons by establishing a fluid deposit with a saline solution beneath the site. This technique was particularly useful in patients with large burns, when skin had to be taken from several sites. Barker (1951) also examined the thickness of the skin at several sites in cadavers. The palpebral skin was found to be the thinnest, with the skin of the postauricular and the inguinal region ranking next. The skin of the back was the thickest. Foreskin is not mentioned in his article.

Because of the improvement in the treatment of shock and better care of the general condition of the patient, larger skin defects from burns or other trauma demanded skin grafts. More and more skin was grafted in a single session. The question arose whether the amount of skin cut in one session should not be restricted in view of the substantial blood loss during this procedure. A study by Robinson (1949) revealed that the cutting of 100 cm^2 skin with a Padgett dermatome involved an average loss of 23 ml blood. The cutting of thicker grafts involved more blood loss than the cutting of thinner grafts. Graft cutting from the back or buttocks involved more blood loss than cutting from other sites such as the abdomen, chest and thighs. Younger patients averaged a larger blood loss than patients over 45. Patients in good nutritional condition lost more blood than those in poor nutritional condition.

This information was important as the expected blood loss could be assessed and preventive measures taken.

Healing of Donor Sites

Several surgeons studied the way in which donor sites healed. The process of re-epithelialization was found to arise from the ectodermal components of the hair follicles and the sebaceous glands; the role of the hair follicles was most prominent in this respect. When grafts had been cut deep into the corium, the epithelial structures of the sweat glands made a greater contribution to re-epithelialization, because the cut had been made below the hair follicles. In donor areas which healed quickly, the epithelium was found to have been formed over a thin layer of loose connective tissue. Elastic fibres did not develop until some time after epithelialization. As late as five weeks after epithelialization of the entire donor area, only very small elastic fibres were found to be present.

The process of re-epithelialization proved to be very vulnerable and any irritation – be it chemical, bacterial or mechanical – delayed or prevented healing so that epithelialization might take as long as 6–8 weeks instead of 10 days.

Converse and Robb-Smith (1944) introduced the concept of "inter-island contraction" with regard to the healing of donor sites. This inter-island contraction meant that epithelial islands unite with adjacent islands not only through cell division and migration but also through contraction. The role of inter-island contraction increased in importance as the time required for epithelialization increased. The donor sites of thin grafts showed only slight contraction (2–5% of the surface area), but the donor sites of thick ones showed more.

Entin et al. (1948) performed an original clinical experiment with skin graft donor sites, to investigate the influence of cold on healing, epithelial regeneration and fibrous tissue formation. The temperature at the wound surface ranged from 11.6° to 27.8 °C. Cooling was continued for 3–13 days. The time required for complete epithelialization of the wounds proved to be inversely proportional to the temperature, and directly proportional to the duration of exposure to cold. Exposure to a temperature of 11.6°–18.3 °C delayed epithelialization by 3–4 days. The rate of epithelialization was more influenced than extra fibrous tissue formation. In the cooled donor areas, the fibrous tissue showed oedema which persisted for several weeks. Based on their experiments, these investigators concluded that the optimal environmental temperature should be between 21.1° and 26.7 °C, and that epithelialization was completed most quickly when the temperature of the wound surface was 32.3°–35 °C. The unfavourable effect of cold on wound healing had been previously studied in the laboratory by Large and Heinbecker (1944), who studied dogs with full-thickness skin loss. The wounds were cooled with water at 4°–8 °C for 24–72 hours. These wounds showed delayed healing, the delay being directly proportional to the duration of cooling.

After-Care of Donor Sites

The donor sites were covered with several types of dressing, e.g. with gauze containing Xeroform, a 5% tannic acid spray (Padgett 1942) or a 2% aqueous solution of tannic acid (Goode 1935). No further dressings were used when a crust had formed. Other investigators used gauze covered with 5% scarlet red ointment (Brown and McDowell 1943) or petrolatum (Conway and Coldwater 1946). Gradually, however, tulle gras [2] was more and more widely used. Experience has probably played an important role in the increasing preference for the application of greased gauze (Brown and McDowell 1943). The theoretical advantages seem to be logical. Lindquist (1946) attempted to discover its significance in wound healing in an experimental study with different types of dressing, e.g. dry dressings, vaselined gauze and lanolined gauze. He found that both epithelialization and wound contraction were slower in wounds covered with dry dressings than in those covered with the other two dressings. As compared with vaselined gauze, the difference in duration of epithelialization was 100%, and the difference in duration of contraction was 30%. The differences from lanolined dressings were less marked: 40% in duration of epithelialization and 40% in duration of contraction.

A compressing bandage on the donor site was generally regarded as promoting wound healing (Entin et al. 1948).

Preservation of Skin Grafts

The question of whether skin grafts could be preserved without destroying their vitality was no longer a purely scientific problem but had assumed practical importance. To begin with, there were situations in which a graft could not be immediately applied, e.g. in view of haemostasis problems (Webster 1944 a). Secondly, it was important to obtain adequate information on possibilities of preservation with a view to the establishment of skin banks (Strumia and Hodge 1945; Matthews 1945). Within a few years, various studies enhanced the insight into these problems.

In 1943, Brown and McDowell observed that little was yet known about the technique and possibilities of preservation. They had stored a full-thickness skin graft in a refrigerator for 48 hours, whereupon the autografts were accepted well. However, their statement that "as far as is known this was the first clinical instance of the use of this procedure" seems not entirely true. As already mentioned in previous chapters, studies of these possibilities had already been made. Contem-

---

2 Tulle gras, first manufactured in France, is fine-meshed curtain net impregnated with vaseline (98 parts), balsam of Peru (1 part) and olive oil or codliver oil (1 part) (Matthews 1943). In 1919, the Dutch surgeon van Eden had already described the technique in the preparation of this type of dressing (van Eden 1919).

poraries had made casual remarks about skin preservation in their publications. One was Ashley (1937), who had stored homografts in physiological saline in a refrigerator (about 4 °C) or packed them in ice cubes. The grafts were kept for a few days to weeks, and were accepted when subsequently applied. Young and Favata (1944) held that grafts could be kept in a refrigerator (about 4 °C) for up to two weeks without problems, as long as dehydration was prevented.

Research into possibilities of preservation focused on two methods

a) Preservation at refrigerator temperature
b) Preservation at a very low temperature.

a) Preservation at refrigerator temperature:

Both methods were discussed in a paper read by Webster (1944 a), who had practical experience with preservation of grafts in the refrigerator (about 4 °C). He wrapped his grafts in pliofilm and several layers of Xeroform- or vaseline-impregnated gauze and stored them for a period of up to 3 weeks. In the course of 12 years he had applied 36 grafts so preserved in the treatment of 23 patients. The autografting was always successful but one graft, stored in Ringer's solution, failed to take. J. S. Davis, who was in the audience when Webster presented his paper, remarked that he used the same method and that in his opinion grafts could be stored in the refrigerator for as long as 5 weeks.

Matthews (1945) reached the conclusion that grafts could be stored even longer. He rolled grafts in tulle gras and moistened gauze, and placed them in a bottle which was then sealed and stored in a refrigerator (3 °–6 °C). Even after 7 months, the split-skin grafts were still entirely intact according to Matthews, and presented an unchanged appearance at macroscopic and microscopic examination. Some cells in the deeper layers of epidermis showed vacuolation. Fragments of the grafts were cultured on chicken plasma and embryo extracts after 8 days' preservation. Fibroblasts began to grow after 8 days, and mitoses were observed after 17 days. Bacteriological examination of the grafts yielded variable findings: some cultures were sterile while others showed growth of a variety of bacteria such as staphylococci and micrococci. Matthews stated that grafts preserved for less than 3 weeks grew more readily on granulating wound surfaces than fresh grafts. Grafts preserved for 3–8 weeks grew as well as fresh grafts on fresh wounds. He assumed that a correlation existed between refrigeration and "power of growth", which made these grafts more resistant to certain pathogens.

Matthews' conclusion prompted Flatt (1948) to investigate the clinical possibilities of grafting refrigerated skin grafts onto infected wounds. In 17 patients with infected, granulating wounds, 50 split-skin autografts (in the form of so-called stamp grafts) were used which had been stored in a refrigerator for 0–68 days. Only three grafts failed to take. Although a brief period of storage gave better acceptance of the grafts, the acceptance of the longer stored grafts was not unsatisfactory. According to Flatt, the experiments showed that stored skin grafts could quite well be used for infected wounds.

Flatt (1950) continued his studies of the consequences of preservation. In skin kept at 0 °C for four days, the epithelial cells were still quite normal; subsequently the thickness of the keratin and the epithelial layer increased gradually. Flatt assumed that cells which survived preservation developed a kind of tissue hunger, as a result of which both intra- and extracellular growth was promoted.

Briggs and Jund (1944) had gained less favourable experience with skin vitality in earlier experiments. Human autografts stored at 0 °C for 5–20 days were grafted after varying intervals. Five-day-old skin was completely accepted. Of the 10-day-old skin grafts, only 50% were accepted. After 14 days, all grafts failed.

b) Preservation at very low temperatures:

In Webster's report (1944), mention was also made of an attempt to preserve skin at a very low temperature. Skin was frozen with the aid of carbon dioxide snow and butyl alcohol, and then stored for 17 days at –72 °C. A subsequent attempt to graft this skin onto its donor failed. Another graft was frozen by the same technique, but in addition was lyophilized under vacuum. Eighty per cent was accepted.

In another study by Briggs and Jund the consequences of the various cooling techniques were investigated. Moistened skin grafts in a sealed tube were cooled to –78.5 °C at different rates of cooling. Some of the grafts were cooled to what they called the critical temperature of 0 ° to –15 °C within 1.75–2.2 minutes; other grafts were so cooled within 2.5–3 minutes, and yet other grafts were first placed in ice-water for 15–35 minutes and then submitted to this procedure. About 50% of all grafts in these three groups showed satisfactory acceptance (duration of observation: 10–21 weeks). The grafts of the last group showed the highest rate of acceptance and Biggs and Jund attributed this not to the pretreatment with ice-water, but to the fact that these grafts had been rewarmed most quickly! They held that relatively slow freezing caused intercellular ice to form first, thus perhaps preventing the freezing of the cells themselves. In their opinion the survival of cells largely depended on their ability to undergo reversible dehydration.

This theory was not accepted by Strumia and Hodge (1945), who held that the physicochemical properties of complex colloids in the cells were probably best preserved by a combination of "rapid" freezing, storage at –15 °C and rapid rewarming to 37 °C. Their hypothesis was tested in the following experiment: grafts were placed in bottles containing 10–15 ml plasma and placed in an environment with a temperature of –20 ° to –25 °C. Complete freezing was effected in 15–30 minutes. After 1–61 days the grafts were rewarmed to 37 °C in a water-bath, and 80% of the 41 grafts used were accepted. They concluded that, in their model, there was no correlation between grafting result and duration of storage.

Application of the Grafts

Efforts were usually made to cover the entire defect with grafts, although some surgeons applied so-called stamp grafts to granulating wounds (Goode 1935; Webster 1944 b; Hardy and McNichol 1944; Flatt 1948; Buff 1952).

The stamp grafting technique was perfected by Gabarro (1943). The enlargement technique he used, enabled him to cover a defect which was 6–9 times as large as the size of the original skin graft. The skin graft was glued onto stiff sticky paper. Graft and paper were then cut into strips, which were glued parallel to each other and regularly spaced onto another sheet of stiff sticky paper. Perpendicular to the previous cuts, new strips were then cut, which in turn were glued onto a new sheet of stiff sticky paper. Surface area enlargement was thus achieved, and as many squares of skin could be cut as were required. [3]

The grafts which covered the entire defect were fixed to the wound edges with a continuous suture or with interrupted sutures. In some cases the graft was sutured onto the underlying structure as well, to ensure firm contact with it. For grafting on granulation tissue, perforations were usually made in the grafts to ensure drainage of blood and serum. This was not done for fresh wounds, nor as a rule for grafts in the face. The grafts were sutured under a certain amount of tension in order to keep the endothelial spaces open (Padgett 1942).

In spite of standardization of this technique, many complications evidently developed. Publications on glueing techniques to ensure better cohesion between graft and wound floor, which appeared in the forties, received much attention (Sano 1943 a, 1943 b; Young and Favata 1944; Young 1944; Cronkite et al. 1944; Davis 1944; Matthews 1945; Branch et al. 1946; Lagrot 1948). A physiological glue was used for this purpose, and the means used did not differ very widely. The technique described by Sano (1943 a) was still rather complicated, but simplifications were soon introduced. Sano used plasma and an extract of solid blood constituents. The undersurface of the graft was painted with the extract, and the wound floor with plasma. Later, the extract was replaced by thrombin which was commercially available (Young and Favata 1944). Fibrin formation produced an aqueous substance which was drained off via perforations in the graft. Although less fluid formed with the combination of thrombin and fibrinogen, the same drainage was effected in this method (Cronkite et al. 1944). "Glueing" was done both with full-thickness and with split-skin grafts (Sano). Cohesion was initially assumed to be sufficiently strong to make graft suturing and compression bandages superfluous (Sano 1943 b; Young and Favata 1944), but this soon proved to be too optimistic.

A study published by Young showed that compressing bandages were an important means to ensure better results. Young even went further: he found the results of "glueing" so disappointing for granulating wounds that he restricted this technique to fresh wounds. Brown, who initially had been a strong advocate of this technique (Brown and McDowell 1943), later retracted (Brown 1944). Several surgeons subsequently reverted to the technique proposed by Sano (Branch et al. 1946; May 1947).

After the introduction of sulpha-drugs and antibiotics, these were locally applied to the wound bed before grafts were applied, or antibiotic solutions were injected between graft and wound floor. The use of antibiotics did not lead to a decrease in the incidence of infection (Padgett 1942; Matthews 1943; Rawles 1945; Baxter 1946; Howes 1947; Tappeiner 1947; Lagrot 1948). Schuchardt (1949) cautioned against too prolonged application of penicillin and streptomycin in view of the risk of formation of a resistant flora.

---

3 This system was subsequently further perfected by Meek (1958, 1963) and given the name "microdermagrafting". The Meek-Wall microdermatome was used for this.

After-Care of the Grafted Area

The compression bandage has already been mentioned several times as an important aid in grafting. American authors in particular stressed this again and again, but British reports attached less importance to it (Brown and McDowell 1943).

The compression bandage was used to restrict the accumulation of blood and serum beneath the graft, and the formation of oedema. This was believed to reduce the risk of infection. The first layer of the dressing usually consisted of fine-mesh gauze which was left dry (Leithauser 1933) or impregnated with a saline solution (Ludwig 1946). Wet dressings were used especially when the wound had initially been infected. The gauze was impregnated with a variety of substances such as merthiolate, Xeroform, sulphadiazin, scarlet red (May 1947) or acetic acid-glycerin-saline solution (Ludwig 1946). In some cases the gauze was greased with vaseline (Goode 1935; Roberts and Schaubel 1945). Later, nearly all types of dressing were superseded by vaseline-impregnated "tulle gras" (Matthews 1943; Buff 1952). This first layer was usually covered with several layers of gauze which were fixed with a bandage or with adhesive plaster. On the gauzes, sponges were sometimes placed which were fastened with bandages (Padgett 1942; Matthews 1943; Conway and Goldwater 1946).

Results of Skin Grafting

The literature shows that it is difficult to record the results of skin grafting. Complete reports on results should consider several factors, e.g. the objective of the graft, the condition of the wound prior to grafting, the dimensions of the wound, the location of the graft, the type of graft and the criteria that should be applied in evaluation.

Publications in which all these factors received due consideration could not be found. The authors usually focused on only one or a few aspects. In the following discussion of the results, the emphasis will be on the restoration of the functions of the grafted skin.

Padgett (1942) was one of the authors who studied graft acceptance. He was aware of the fact that an evaluation of acceptance gave no information on the long-term result (contraction). Thin grafts (by his own criteria 0.2–0.25 mm thick) nearly always showed 100% acceptance on "aseptic denuded surfaces". However, the features of the integument (e.g. colour) deteriorated with the passage of time. A 50%–70% contraction of the thin grafts was not unusual. Padgett obtained better results with three-quarter-thickness skin grafts on aseptic denuded surfaces. The mean take of this type of graft, used on 137 patients, was 96%. Padgett added that this finding as such was inconclusive because all cases in which the take was not complete had to be regarded as complete failures. Three-quarter-thickness skin grafts applied to a substructure as loose as that in the cervical region showed 10%–35% contraction. This did not exceed the rate of contraction of full-thickness skin grafts under similar conditions. The long-term results achieved with three-quarter-thickness skin grafts did not differ from those achieved with full-thickness grafts.

The acceptance results reported by Conway and Goldwater (1946) seem to be much less favourable. They worked on war victims under wartime conditions, in military hospitals far from home and their objective was to close the defects as quickly as possible with the simplest means available. They achieved complete acceptance with 86.6% of 306 grafts, partial acceptance with 6.9% and complete failure with 6.5%. It is to be noted that 35% of all operations were performed by novices. The principal causes of failure were: errors in assessing bacterial contamination, inadequate or wrong planning, and insufficient immobilization.

Brown and McDowell (1942 a, 1943) likewise recognized the problems involved in establishing the criteria of a good result. They held that a result could be described as good if:

a) Sufficient skin was available for unimpaired movement
b) The cicatrix was reasonably flexible
c) Trauma sustained in day-to-day activities caused no damage
d) Sensibility was normal.

They added, however, that even if this functional result was obtained the cosmetic result could be (and often was) disappointing. The disappointing cosmetic results of facial skin grafts prompted them to use local flaps as often as possible for facial defects. However, with local flaps, too, there remained conspicuous differences in colour. Byars (1945) therefore decided to adjust the colour of facial flaps or grafts by tattooing. The 60 patients he treated all showed improvement of appearance.

In discussing their results, Brown and McDowell (1943) repeatedly mentioned that both split-skin grafts and full-thickness grafts used on children increased in size during growth. They were unable to explain this "growth" mechanism, and also found it difficult to explain contractures which developed as a complication after grafting. Perhaps an infection deep in the wound bed might play a role in this respect. Their experience was that keloid formation occurred mostly in small, obese girls. Surface irradiation (which was occasionally proposed as therapy) had not had the desired effect in any of these patients. Another complication mentioned by Brown and McDowell consisted of an accumulation of sebum beneath the grafts. This was observed in particular with thick split-skin grafts. It might perhaps be explained by retrograde secretion of sebum from the cut glands. The accumulation of sebum, which occurred after 3–4 weeks, sometimes unfavourably influenced the grafting result, particularly if infection developed. They therefore advocated the earliest possible removal of the sebum by pressure, if necessary combined with incisions.

Restoration of Sensibility

Research into restoration of sensibility started after 1930, and initially focused mainly on sensibility in pedicled flaps (Kredel and Evans 1933; Davis 1934; Davis and Kitlovski 1934; Hutchison et al. 1949; McGregor 1950). Restoration of sensibility in free skin grafts received less attention. In other review articles, restoration of sensibility was discussed only superficially (Garlock 1933; Brown and McDowell 1941, 1943).

Garlock held that a zone of hyperaesthesia formed around full-thickness skin grafts and persisted for some time. Tactile sensibility recovered first in the grafts, and extended from the periphery to the centre. He observed the first signs of recovery of sensibility 6 weeks after grafting. After tactile sensibility, pain sense and temperature sense recovered. In small and medium-sized grafts (exact dimensions were not specified), sensibility was restored completely within 6 months. In large grafts this took a year or longer.

One of the first systematic studies of recovery of sensibility, chiefly in pedicled flaps, was that published by Kredel and Evans in 1933. They considered the questions whether, to what extent, and in what order the various qualities of sensibility were restored. On the basis of their findings in a small group of patients they concluded that sensibility was best restored in pedicled flaps. Virtually all subsequent investigators agreed with this conclusion. The full-thickness skin graft ranked next in quality of recovery. Pain sense, however, did not fully return even after 3–5 years, and tactile sensibility was in fact still completely absent. Pinch grafts, studied in 5 patients, showed even poorer restoration of sensibility. The least favourable results were obtained with split-skin grafts: there was some recovery of pain sense after 8–18 months in four of the five grafts, but sensibility recovered only in patches. Pain sense returned first in the grafts, followed by tactile sensibility and finally by temperature sense.

The findings obtained by L. Davis largely agreed with those described by Kredel and Evans. Sensibility was usually restored only in patches, within 4–5 weeks in the most favourable cases but in most patients much later (sometimes years later). The type of graft and the presence of cicatricial tissue around and beneath the graft were factors which Kredel and Evans had also mentioned. A few years later a publication by McCaroll (1938) caused some sensation because it attacked more or less established views. McCaroll examined a large group of children 5–15 years after operative treatment with the aid of pedicled flaps, full-thickness and split-skin grafts. He studied pain sense, tactile sensibility and two-point discrimination. Recovery of temperature sense was such as to warrant no conclusions for pedicled flaps or full-thickness and split-skin grafts. He did a follow-up over a 3-year period in 45 patients who had received split-skin grafts. In these patients sensibility first returned in scattered areas, and was completely restored within a short time thereafter, usually within 60 days. Pain sense and tactile sensibility returned completely all through the split-skin grafts. The best results with split-skin grafts were obtained on a fresh wound bed with a substructure of virtually normal tissue after excision of thin scars. Results of grafts in areas with abundant cicatricial tissue were much less good. Grafts applied directly to muscle tissue showed slow restoration of sensibility. Full-thickness skin grafts showed less early recovery of sensibility than split-skin grafts. In the children this restoration occurred much more quickly than other investigators had observed. The temporal dissociation in return of pain and touch was much greater in full-thickness skin grafts than in split-skin grafts.

McCaroll's findings received little credit. Padgett (1942) was among the few who accepted his conclusions. Some of Padgett's patients in fact showed return of pain sense in split-skin grafts within 20 days, with complete restoration of sensibility within 60 days.

Doubts about McCaroll's findings prompted Kernwein (1948) to reduplicate the study on 74 (free) skin grafts with 95%–100% take in all cases. Some of the grafts had been used to cover defects resulting from the transfer of pedicled flaps. The area of these donor sites showed a normal anatomy. Kernwein observed that sensibility returned in patches, which gradually increased in size. The pain threshold gradually diminished in the centre of the patches. Nevertheless, large areas in the graft remained in which no pain could be perceived. Under favourable conditions, sensibility in split-skin grafts returned in patches within 7–9 weeks. The best results were observed in grafts which had been used to cover donor sites of pedicled flaps; nearly complete recovery of sensibility occurred in these grafts.

All investigators agreed that growth of nerve fibres around and beneath the grafts was seriously impeded by cicatricial tissue. Kredel and Evans (1933) and Davis (1934) assumed that nerve fibres grew from tissues around and beneath the grafts. Kernwein (1948) held that nerve fibres only grew from the undersurface of the grafts.

Subsequently, research into return of sensibility in grafts was more or less dormant for a long time, but in 1959 and 1960 important contributions were published and, although these fell outside the period under discussion here, they will be discussed in order to complete the survey, as was mentioned in the preface.

The Dutch investigators Sneep, Folkerts and Meyling (1959) studied return of sensibility in split-skin grafts after early excision of burns and after secondary, delayed grafting. After early excision and grafting, sensibility proved to return almost completely. The pattern of sensibility in the graft corresponded with that in the surrounding skin. After secondary, delayed grafting, return of sensibility was much less complete. Histological examination with a view to the presence of nerve tissue confirmed this. Much more nerve tissue had grown in the grafts applied after early excision. Sneep and his collaborators concluded that regeneration of nerve tissue was determined by the time lag between the injury and the moment of grafting; the thickness and type of graft were of much less importance in this respect.

Shortly after the monograph of Sneep et al. was published, Pontén (1960) published a study in which return of sensibility was discussed in equal detail. Pontén confined his study to grafts applied under favourable conditions, usually in patients with burns. Some 50% of the split-skin grafts were applied to wounds which were a few weeks or months old. In some patients the first sign of returning sensibility was hyperaesthesia in the grafts.

Tactile sensibility ultimately returned to normal in all patients. In several patients the pain threshold in the grafts was diminished. Like Sneep, Pontén concluded that in grafts showing adequate reinnervation, tactile sensibility finally equalled that of adjacent skin. All grafts showed good recovery of temperature sense. The two-point discrimination tests showed that sensibility resumed the same pattern as that in adjacent skin. There was no difference between the various types of graft, although tactile sensibility seemed to return more readily in full-thickness skin grafts (Pontén 1960). Pontén considered the two-point discrimination test to be the most relevant yardstick of graft reinnervation.

Restoration of the Function of the Sweat Glands

Not much has been published on recovery of sympathetic functions in grafted skin. One of the first studies devoted to this subject was published by Kredel and Phemister (1939), who examined two split-skin grafts and one full-thickness skin graft, focusing mainly on the question whether they had recovered their ability to perspire. The full-thickness skin graft partly recovered this ability, but the other grafts did not (not even more than 5 years after grafting).

A study by Conway (1939) likewise focused on recovery of the ability to perspire. Small deep grafts were found to perspire normally and full-thickness skin grafts could also be made to sweat; but this was possible with only two of 15 split-skin grafts. Conway concluded that recovery of the ability to perspire depended on the presence of sweat glands in the graft. He was unable to answer the question whether sympathetic nerve fibres had to recover before sweating was possible.

The previously mentioned study by Pontén revealed that grafts in which sensibility was permanently disturbed contained no functioning sweat glands. If the sweat glands did function, they assumed the pattern of perspiration of the surrounding skin. The sweat glands were hypersensitive to electrophoretic stimulation with nicotine sulphate.

Restoration of the Function of the Sebaceous Glands

In Pontén's monograph, recovery of the function of the sebaceous glands in various graft types was also examined. Full-thickness skin grafts produced the same amount of ether-soluble substance (sebum) as comparable skin. The amount of ether-soluble substance in split-skin grafts was less than that in a comparable skin area. However, the sum of the amounts of ether-soluble sebum in the split-skin graft and its donor area exceeded the amount in a comparable skin area. Functioning sebaceous glands were found in split-skin grafts. The activity of these glands was unrelated to the sensibility in the grafts. The presence of functioning pilomotor muscles in the grafts was not required for discharge of the sebum.

Changes in Pigmentation

Most authors recorded colour differences which had developed in grafts, but they were unable to explain the phenomenon. Padgett (1942) held that intensified pigmentation in grafts occurred especially in brunettes, but not in true blondes. He observed pigment changes mostly in grafts whose superficial layer had become detached during acceptance. The pattern of pigmentation remained unchanged in grafts accepted without vesiculation.

According to Brown and McDowell (1943), the tension on the graft sutures and subsequent contraction (if any) played a role in the change of pigmentation in that they caused a change in the number of pigment granules per unit of surface area. According to Pontén (1960), the donor site was also important in this respect: the larger the distance between donor site and grafting site, the more marked the differences in pigmentation that could be expected.

Experiments failed to produce much information on the background of pigment changes. The possibilities of experimental investigation seemed limited.

One of the few attempts at experimental research was made by Fessler (1941) who studied the question of whether the ability of the melanoblasts to form melanin could be influenced by the environment (grafting) in spotted guinea-pigs. Pigmented split-skin grafts with a diameter of 3–4 mm were taken from an animal and transferred to a non-pigmented area of the same animal's skin. The epidermis regenerated within 3 weeks. Pigment granules were found in the cells of the basement layer, but cells with melanin were found also in the epidermis of the initially non-pigmented area. Non-pigmented grafts applied to wounds in pigmented areas degenerated. A new epidermis with scattered pigment cells developed 8–10 days after grafting. Fessler (1941) reached the remarkable conclusion that, in guinea-pigs, non-pigmented skin grafts behaved like homografts when applied to a wound in a pigmented skin area. He assumed that melanoblasts had a higher degree of vitality and a more marked growth potential than other epithelial cells. He thought it conceivable that the potential of these melanoblasts for super-regeneration was stimulated by the change of environment (grafting).

Healing of Grafts

After 1930, several aspects of graft acceptance also continued to be studied. Billingham and Reynolds (1953), for example, published an original study of the behaviour of pure epidermal grafts in rabbits. The grafts were obtained as described by Medawar (1941): trypsin powder in a Tyrode solution which contained phenol red was used to remove the corium from split-skin grafts. The grafts were immersed in this solution for one hour at a temperature of 37 °C, and this caused the elastic fibres to dissolve so that the cohesion between epidermis and corium disappeared. Medawar himself had already suggested that this technique could be used in experiments with epithelial sheets.

Ten days after grafting of the epidermis, the epithelium was found to show marked hyperplasia. The thickness of the entire epithelial layer had increased to 90–120 μm. There seemed to be adequate cohesion between epithelium and wound bed. The granulation tissue extended beneath the epithelium. Although after 25 days the epithelium still showed marked proliferative activity, the vital epithelial layer could be detached in its entirety from the underlying structure after the 16th day.

Microscopic examination showed that the epithelial protrusions on the undersurface of the grafts had disappeared. According to Billingham and Reynolds, this corroborated Szodoray's postulate (1931) that elastic fibres play an important role in the cohesion between epidermis and corium. In the pure epidermal grafts, these elastic fibres were no longer present. The experiments were repeated with pure epidermal cell grafts and revealed that the epidermal cell suspension showed about the same reaction as the sheets. Within 16 days the epithelial islets merged to form a single unit, but this epithelial integument did not prevent contraction of the wound bed.

Billingham and Reynolds (1953) also concluded from these experiments that epithelium alone was an insufficient cover for wounds. Corium was required for an adequate integument. The ideal cell suspension should contain mesenchymal elements as well as epithelial cells; it could then become an adequate corium substitute by cellular proliferation and formation of fibrous tissue.

Rous (1946) published an article with the promising title "The activation of skin grafts". It described grafting experiments in rabbits, made in order to establish whether the grafts could be stimulated so as to take more quickly. Before cutting the grafts, the donor site was painted with a mixture of turpentine and acetone, or with chloroform, and the inflammatory reaction thickened the epidermis. Grafts from such sites took more quickly and showed more rapid epithelialization. The donor site, too, healed more quickly than did control areas. Rous conceded that this method could entail some risk for human patients in view of the toxic effects of turpentine and chloroform. In fact he wrote: "It may well be that activation will remain a principle, not become a practicality."

The lymph flow in grafts was studied by McGregor and Conway (1956) with the aid of a contrast medium injected into the corium of the graft. On the 6th day after grafting this contrast medium usually drained readily from the graft, and the graft oedema diminished when the lymph circulation was restored.

In the fifties, histochemical studies of skin grafts also commenced. For example, glycogen and RNA concentrations were determined (Scothorne and Tough 1952; Scothorne and Scothorne 1953). This was done because glycogen and RNA were regarded as representative for the carbohydrate and the protein metabolism. Glycogen was demonstrable in biopsy specimens from grafts two days after grafting; after five days it was present in abundant amounts. Normal skin was found to contain but little glycogen. Glycogen concentration in autografts remained unchanged up to the 20th day.

In homografts it decreased after 15 days because the epithelial cells disintegrated; the epithelial cells which remained intact still contained glycogen. In view of the high concentration of glycogen in the epithelial cells, it was considered unlikely that homografts disintegrated due to inability to produce glycogen. Prior to the degeneration of the cells in the homografts, no marked increase or decrease in glycogen concentration occurred.

The questions which remained unanswered were why the glycogen concentration in epithelial cells increased after grafting, and where the glycogen came from. Was there adaptation to a state of hypoxia?

Cytoplasmic basophils were regarded as indicators of RNA. Up to the 4th day after grafting, the RNA concentration was still low. Subsequently the concentration increased, and cytoplasmic basophils increased along with a thickening of the epidermis due to cellular proliferation and increased cell size. After 20 days, the mitotic activity and the size of the cells in autografts returned to normal. In homografts, the RNA concentration decreased after 10 days, probably due to destruction of cells.

B. Full-Thickness Skin Grafts

Indications

There were fewer indications for full-thickness skin grafting than for split-skin grafting. The fact that great technical skill and an ideal wound floor were required limited the range of indications (Garlock 1933; Dufourmentel 1939). Yet views on the principal applications differed. Some considered these grafts most suitable for the extremities, near joints (Garlock 1933; Brown and McDowell 1943). Others regarded them as particularly useful for reconstructions in the face, e.g. for eyelids, eyebrows, around the nose and the mouth (Dufourmentel 1937; Padgett 1942; Brown and Cannon 1945). It was agreed almost unanimously that full-thickness skin grafts were very suitable for the hands (Garlock 1933; Dufourmentel 1937; Koch 1941; Padgett 1942; Brown and McDowell 1943; May 1947).

The indications most frequently mentioned were congenital or acquired (burns) contractures, webbed fingers, syndactyly, Dupuytren's contracture and radiation dermatitis without ulceration. Generally, full-thickness skin grafts were only used for fresh wounds of limited dimensions.

Grafting Technique

The Donor Site

The inside of the upper arm or thigh was much less often used than previously (Brown and McDowell 1943). One of the principal reasons was that larger defects were covered with split-skin grafts or, if necessary, with three-quarter-thickness skin grafts. If a large full-thickness skin graft was required, it was taken from the abdominal wall or the inguinal region (Dragstedt and Wilson 1937; Dufourmentel 1937, 1939). The back was no longer used as a donor site.

The most popular donor sites were the retroauricular area (Dufourmentel 1937, 1939; Byars 1945; Buff 1952) or the supraclavicular region (Brown and Cannon 1945; Byars 1945; Buff 1952), because the colour of the skin at these sites matches that of the face, and the skin contains little subcutis. The retroauricular area had the additional advantage that the scar at this site remained invisible. Foreskin and labial skin were hardly used.

Graft-Cutting Technique

The shape of the graft required was marked on the skin in various colours and a graft of the same size as the defect to be covered, or slightly larger, was carefully dissected out (Iselin 1945). As a rule, the skin was then carefully lifted and stretched with a retractor or some other instrument, and separated from the subcutis (Burian 1937; Brown and McDowell 1943; Buff 1952).

Shafiroff (1935) was among the few who tried to use a specific instrument in dissecting full-thickness skin grafts. The instrument consisted of a punch mounted on a syringe (Fig. 43); a local anaesthetic could be injected through a needle centred in the punch.

After excision of the graft, the donor site was generally closed with sutures. Brown and McDowell (1943) were perhaps an exception: they allowed the wound to heal by second intention or, if the defect was large, applied a split-skin graft to it.

Application of Grafts and After-Care

Dufourmentel (1937) urged that the grafts should be applied as quickly as possible in order to prevent loss of temperature and dehydration. The grafts were sutured under normal tension, either with a continuous suture (Garlock 1933) or with interrupted sutures (Brown and Cannon 1945). In some cases, deep mattress sutures were passed through graft and substructure to ensure additional fixation. Only exceptionally were perforations made in the grafts for drainage of blood or serum.

Dragstedt and Wilson (1937) and Burian (1937) made multiple parallel overlapping incisions in full-thickness skin grafts. Not only did this ensure adequate drainage but it also enabled them to place the grafts in any desired pattern (concertina effect) and to cover a surface area twice or three times as large as the original graft (mesh principle).

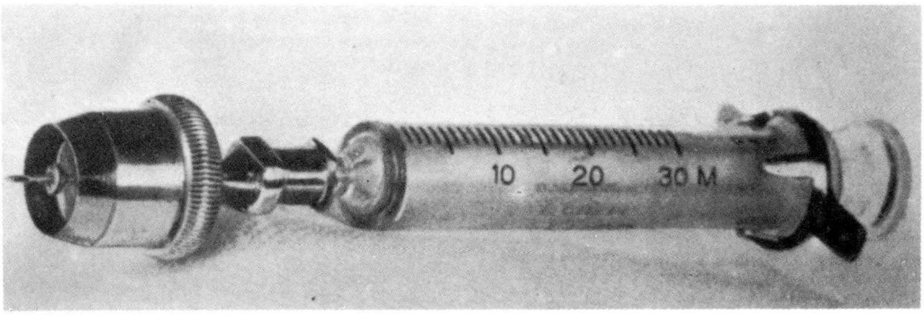

Fig. 43. An instrument to cut full-thickness skin grafts designed by Shafiroff (1935)

The grafted wound was dressed in about the same way as wounds with split-skin grafts. A dry or greased gauze was placed on the graft, and initially a sponge was placed on top of this gauze (Garlock). Subsequently, several layers of gauze were used instead of a sponge. Mould fixation was applied at sites where conventional dressings gave insufficient compression and immobilization. Nearly all authors considered a firm compression bandage essential. After grafting on extremities, additional immobilization was effected with the aid of splints (plaster of Paris, crinoline or wood).

Mention should be made of a remark which MacFee (1933) made in a discussion of a paper read by Garlock (1933). MacFee advised burying full-thickness skin grafts beneath adjacent tissues in order to ensure an optimal take: in this way, the epithelial part of the graft could perhaps obtain some nutrition from the tissues on top of it!

Dressings were usually left in situ for about 8–10 days (Garlock 1933; Burian 1937; Dufourmentel 1937; May 1947). Brown and McDowell (1943) made an exception for grafts around the eyes, nose and mouth; at these sites the dressings were changed after 5 days because they were moist as a result of secretion. Dressings and splints continued to be used for up to three weeks after grafting. During the first six weeks after grafting, the graft was protected as far as possible from mechanical injuries (Garlock 1933).

Infections were combatted with various disinfectant fluids, e.g. boric acid wet dressing. In some cases, necrotic tissue in grafts was excised as soon as possible and the defects were painted with 10% merbromin solution (Brown and McDowell 1943).

Results

Many continued to be intrigued by the question why the slight difference in thickness between a split-skin graft and a full-thickness skin graft made such a difference in long-term contraction. Brown and McDowell (1943) observing that contraction arose from the wound floor suggested that the cut hair follicles and sweat glands irritated the under-surface of split skin grafts, thus causing irritation of the wound bed and consequently more marked cicatrization. Opinions on the severity of contraction of full-thickness skin grafts differed. Some authors assumed that, after a perfect take, there was no contraction at all (Garlock 1933). Like split-skin grafting, full-thickness skin grafting was sometimes followed by marked changes in pigmentation.

The results in terms of restoration of functions, such as sensibility, have been discussed earlier in this chapter.

C. Homografting

It has been described in previous chapters how clinical experience and experimental findings had shown that skin homografting was bound to fail. Nevertheless, for years a number of surgeons continued to believe in this type of grafting (Roegholt 1976). In the thirties there were still several publications reporting good results of homografting, e.g. with foreskin (Ashley 1937; Sachs and Goldberg 1943). The influence of compatibility of blood groups between donor and recipient on homografting results was also re-studied by Binhold in 1939. Binhold (1939) concluded that 50% of the homografts were accepted, regardless of blood group compatibility, 20% of these homografts degenerated later, 30% led to permanent success.

A few years after Binhold's publication, Gibson and Medawar (1943) suggested that the results were probably based on misinterpretation. Binhold had used very small grafts, which were probably absorbed very gradually, with cicatrization caused by epithelium from the wound edges.

The small group of advocates of homografting gradually diminished, as demonstrated in publications by the renowned French plastic surgeon Dufourmentel. Initially he reported that, in a small group of patients, he had observed no differences between the results of autografting and those of homografting; however, donor and recipient should have the same blood group (Dufourmentel 1933 a, b). In the first edition of his book *Chirurgie réparatrice et correctrice,* Dufourmentel stated in 1939 that, although homografting had become obsolete, he nevertheless still saw some indications for it. The homografts were partly absorbed after a while, but the remaining vestiges of corium could, he believed, play an important role in epithelialization. In the second edition of his book (1950), Dufourmentel retracted all previous positive statements about homografting.

Successful Homografting in Monozygotic Twins

Homografting in monozygotic twins was a challenge to many surgeons, who sometimes waited for years for an apportunity to perform this operation. Bauer

(1927) was probably the first to do so. In the operative correction of syndactyly in twins, he used grafts from one of the children on both patients. The grafts were accepted and retained their functions.

Brown (1937) had also long been looking forward to performing a homograft on identical twins. Finally, male identical twins made themselves available for that experiment. A full-thickness skin graft was obtained from each twin and grafted on the other. Both grafts showed complete and permanent survival.

Padgett (1942) reported on successful grafting in four twins in his monograph; Schattner (1944) and Converse and Duchet (1947) each reported on one pair of twins.

The most dramatic description of homografting in identical twins was undoubtedly that published by McIndoe and Franceschetti (1949). This homografting was used as forensic evidence that two children, brought up by different parents, were in fact twins. The parents of 6-year-old twins were surprised at the resemblance between one of their twins and another child in their neighbourhood. Their surprise increased when they heard that this child had been born in the same hospital as their twins, and on the same day. The father was so obsessed with these similarities that he contacted the authorities and raised the question whether one of his twins could have been inadvertently exchanged. An inquiry was instituted. Reciprocal skin grafting was performed in an effort to clinch the evidence that an exchange had indeed taken place. The exchanged full-thickness graft took in the true twin, and was still present 10 months later. The court then decided that the parents had to exchange the children because one of the pair of twins had been mistaken for another child in the hospital.

New Applications

Several surgeons, particularly in the United States, pointed out that skin homografts could play a useful role as biological dressing, even though they disintegrated in the long run (Brown 1937; Bettman 1938; Brown and McDowell 1942 a, b, 1943; Davis 1934; Webster 1944 a).

The value of homografts as temporary integument was illustrated by Brown (1937) on the basis of the case histories of two patients with large skin defects, to which skin from the mother was applied. The children's general condition thereupon rapidly improved and the critical phase in treatment was overcome. Homografts as skin dressing proved to be extremely useful in particular in patients with large burns.

Bettman (1938) pointed out that, after application of homografts, the patient's body temperature fell, pulse and respiration improved, and the leucocyte count diminished. Most impressive were the improved sense of well-being, increased appetite and vigour, and an improved mental attitude. In patients whose condition was too poor for operative treatment, split-skin homografts were applied. In patients with large burns the process of spontaneous disintegration took 3–10 weeks. Once the patients were restored to a good condition, autografting was done and the remnants of the homografts were removed, if necessary.

Research into Failure of Homografting

Loeb's hypothesis (1930) that homografting was bound to fail, due to interindividual differences, was accepted by most surgeons as a starting-point for further theories. Padgett (1932, 1942) assumed that the homograft released substances which acted as toxins and caused a leucocyte and fibroblast reaction in the recipient. Brown and McDowell (1942 b, 1943) proceeded from the assumption that proteins in the homograft had an antigenic effect, which in the course of three weeks could elicit a maximal allergic reaction in the recipient. In their opinion, skin should be regarded as an organ – not merely as epithelial tissue – and could no more grow and survive in a foreign organism than any other organ.

Histological Findings

Clinical observations on what happened to a homograft sometimes proved to be unreliable. With the aid of the microscope, a more accurate impression could be gained of the changes which occurred. For a long time, interpretation of these processes posed problems because rejection reactions were not understood. It was usually stressed that the presence of interstitial oedema in the homografts caused increased infiltration of round cells and polynuclear cells (Brown and McDowell 1942 a, b, 1943).

The cells of the basement layer of the epidermis lost cohesion, both with each other and with the collagen. The collagenous fibres were infiltrated by polymorphous cells. Slight fibroblastic activity could be observed in the wound surface. A biopsy specimen taken 36 days after homografting was found to contain only a few vestiges of cellular debris. The corium was overgrown by granulation tissue.

Gibson (Fig. 44) and Medawar, in a combined study from the departments of surgery and pathology of the Royal Infirmary in Glasgow, reached in 1943 the conclusion that homografts evidently rapidly caused a reaction of mesenchymal cells and vessels. This reaction diminished before the epidermis completely disappeared, and while the corium was till intact. The collagenous fibres proved to be highly resistant. The biopsy specimens which they examined still contained some collagen even after 36 days. Only in a late phase did erosion of the fibres occur, probably due to histiocytes and other mesenchymal cells. The cuticle cells were found to provoke a multinucleate giant cell reaction. The epidermis disappeared completely between the 10th and the 15th days. Epithelial cells still present after this period showed degenerative characteristics which originated from the basement layer of the epidermis.

The degeneration of epithelium was evidently caused by a humoral mechanism, which Gibson and Medawar interpreted as an immunity reaction. Epithelial degeneration was not accompanied by a local reaction of lymphocytes or other mesenchymal cells. Perhaps a relatively inert material such as collagen could provoke a cellular reaction.

In the course of the study, a second set of homografts (also in the form of pinch grafts) was applied to the same patient. These grafts, however, did not undergo the same cycle of growth and regression as the homografts of the first set. Primary adhesion was much less marked, and there was no growth of epithelium from the

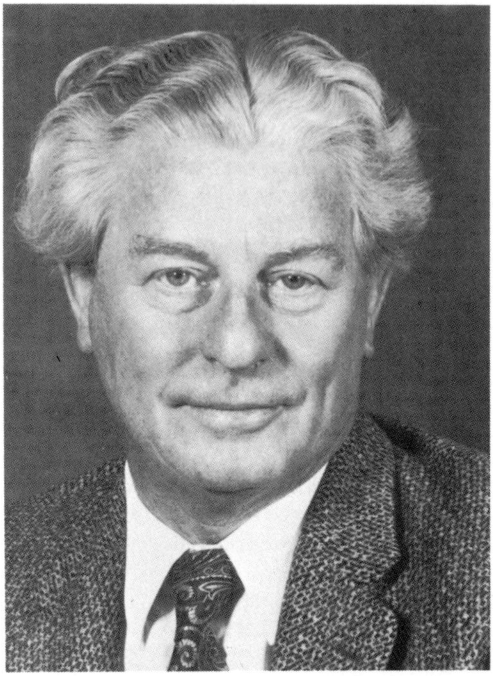

Fig. 44. Tom Gibson, distinguished researcher in the field of homograft wound healing

grafts. The degenerative changes developed at an earlier stage and were more marked than in the first set of homografts. The microscopic features of the second set after 8 days corresponded with those of the first set after 23 days. Gibson and Medawar concluded from this accelerated reaction that the first set of homografts had provoked active immunization.

Medawar (1943, 1944, 1945) continued the experiments with homografts in animals, in an effort to find an answer to the question of whether there was a correlation between the amount of skin grafted and the recipient's reaction to it. One group of rabbits received a relatively large amount of skin (0.34–0.44 g per rabbit), while another group received relatively little (0.006–0.06 g per rabbit). The grafts were accepted in the usual way, but after a phase of hyperplasia acute inflammatory symptoms developed, associated with proliferation of vessels and lymphocytes. The grafts became necrotic after an invasion of lymphocytes and monocytes. In animals which had received a small amount of skin, the median survival time (defined as the time in which 50% of the foreign epithelium degenerated) was 5 days longer than in animals which had received a large amount of skin. A second set of homografts, applied 16 days after the first set, had an average survival time which was about 4 days shorter than that after grafting a large amount of skin in the first set. When the homografts of the second set were applied to the same site as those of the first set, degeneration was slightly quicker than when the second set homografts were applied elsewhere, but the difference was not so marked as to warrant the conclusion that the local immunity conditions contributed to the systemic reaction.

According to Medawar (1945), experiments in which skin was grafted on several sites in the rabbit also demonstrated that rejection of homografts was a systemic reaction. The various homografts were rejected as quickly as the same amount of skin applied to a single site.

In other experiments, Medawar demonstrated that skin from young individuals had equally marked antigenic properties as skin from fully grown individuals (the conviction that the opposite was true had in the past been a reason for grafting skin from foetuses). Other experiments revealed that homografts which filled an entire defect and formed no epithelium survived longer than homografts which were able to form an epithelial zone. The latter were rejected more quickly because the amount of foreign tissue increased cumulatively.

References

Allen HS, Koch SL (1942) The treatment of patients with severe burns. Surg Gynecol Obstet 74:914–924

Ashley F (1937) Foreskins as skin grafts. Ann Surg 106:252–256

Aufricht G, Dowd JF (1948) A mirror attachment on the Padgett's dermatome as a visual guide. Plast Reconstr Surg 3:89–91

Barker DE (1948 a) New donor areas in skin grafting. Ann Surg 127:410–412

Barker DE (1948 b) Vacuotome – a new machine for obtaining split thickness skin grafts. Plast Reconstr Surg 3:492–501

Barker DE (1948 c) Throw-away blades for the dermatome. Plast Reconstr Surg 3:748–749

Barker DE (1950) Cutting skin grafts with the vacuotome. Plast Reconstr Surg 5:188–192

Barker DE (1951) Skin thickness in the human. Plast Reconstr Surg 7:115–116

Bauer KH (1927) Homoiotransplantation von Epidermis bei eineiigen Zwillingen. Bruns' Beitr Klin Chir 141:442–447

Baxter H (1946) The effect of penicillin and streptomycin applied locally on the take of skin grafts. Plast Reconstr Surg 1:322

Berkow SG (1945) Tape method of skin-grafting. US Nav Med Bull 45:1

Bettman AG (1938) Homogenous Thiersch grafting as a life saving measure. Am J Surg 39:156–162

Billingham RE, Reynolds J (1952) Transplantation studies on sheets of pure epidermal epithelium and on epidermal cell suspensions. Br J Plast Surg 5:25–36

Binhold (1939) Ueber homöoplastische Transplantationen menschlicher Haut unter besonderer Berücksichtigung der Blutmerkmale. Dtsch Z Chir 252:183–196

Bodenham DC (1949) A new type of knife for cutting skin grafts, using replaceable blades. Br J Plast Surg 2:136–137

Branch CD, Wilkins GF Ross FP (1946) The coagulum contact method (Sano) of skin grafting in the treatment of burns and wounds. Surgery 19:460–466

Braun W (1934) Hautpfropfung. Zentralbl Chir 61:1296

Briggs R, Jund L (1944) Successful grafting of frozen and thawed mouse skin. Anat Rec 89:75–85

Brown HM (1948) A motor driven dermatome. Ind Med Surg 17:46

Brown JB (1937) Homografting of skin: with report of success in identical twins. Surgery 1:558–563

Brown JB (1944) Discussion: Skin graft fixation by plasma-thrombin adhesion (Young). Ann Surg 120:461

Brown JB McDowell F (1941) Persistence of function of skin grafts through long periods of growth. Surg Gynecol Obstet 72:848–853

Brown JB, McDowell F (1942 a) Epithelial healing and the transplantation of skin. Ann Surg 115:1166–1181

Brown JB, McDowell F (1942 b) Massive repairs of burns with thick split skingrafts: Emergency dressings with homografts. Ann Surg 115:658–674
Brown JB, McDowell F (1943) Skin grafting of burns. Lippincott, Philadelphia
Brown JB, Cannon B (1945) Full-thickness skin grafts from the neck for function and color in eyelid and face repairs. Ann Surg 121:639
Browne HR (1941) Marjolin's ulcer. Am J Surg 54:466–471
Buff HU (1952) Hautplastiken. Thieme, Stuttgart
Burian Fr (1937) The experience of the Prague Institute for Plastic Surgery with free whole thickness skin grafts. Rev Chir Structive 4:264–266
Byars LT (1945) Tattooing of free skin grafts and pedicle flaps. Ann Surg 121:644–648
Cannon PR, Wissler RW, Woolridge RL, Benditt EP (1944) The relationship of protein deficiency to surgical infection. Ann Surg 120:514–525
Clery AB (1950) Simple device to facilitate split-skin grafting. Br J Plast Surg 2:290
Converse JM, Duchet G (1947) Successful homologous skin grafting in a war burn using an identical twin as donor. Plast Reconstr Surg 2:342
Converse JM, Robb-Smith AHT (1944) The healing of surface cutaneous wounds: Its analogy with the healing of superficial burns. Ann Surg 120:873–885
Conway H (1939) Sweating function of transplanted skin. Surg Gynecol Obstet 69:756–761
Conway H, Coldwater KB (1946) Principles in reparative plastic surgery, experiences in general hospital in tropics. Surgery 19:437–459
Cronkite EP, Lozner EL, Deaver JM (1944) Use of thrombin and fibrinogen in skin grafting. JAMA 124:976–978
Davis JS (1944) Discussion: Skin graft fixation by plasma-thrombin adhesion (Young). Ann Surg 120:459
Davis JS, Kitlowski EA (1934) Regeneration of nerves in skin grafts and skin flaps. Am J Surg 24:501
Davis L (1934) The return of sensation to transplanted skin. Surg Gynecol Obstet 59: 533–543
Dragstedt LR, Wilson H (1937) A modified sieve graft; a full thickness skin graft for covering large defects. Surg Gynecol Obstet 65:104–106
Dufourmentel L (1933 a) Les auto, homo, et hétero-greffes en chirurgie réparatrice. Bull Soc Chir Paris 25:269–282
Dufourmentel L (1933 b) Greffe totale homoplastique d'un vaste lambeau cutané. Bull Soc Chir Paris 25:724–726
Dufourmentel L (1937) La practique des greffes libres de peau totale. Bull Soc Chir Paris 29:306–317
Dufourmentel L (1939) Chirurgie réparatrice et correctrice des téguments et des formes. Masson, Paris
Dufourmentel L (1950) Chirurgie réparatrice et correctrice des téguments et des formes. Masson, Paris
van Eden PH (1919) Zalfgaas (Vaseline gauze) in Dutch. Tijdschr Ongev Geneesk 4:341
Entin MA, Baxter H, More RH (1948) Experimental and clinical studies of reduced temperature in injury and repair in man. Plast Reconstr Surg 3:11
Esser JFS (1916) Neue Wege für Chirurgische Plastiken durch Heranziehung der Zahnärztliche Technik. Bruns Beitr Klin Chir 103:547
Eymer H (1935) Instrument zur mechanischen Gewinnung grösserer Thiersch'scher Lappen. Dtsch Med Wochenschr 61:1954–1955
Fessler A (1941) Pigmentation and transplantation. Br J Dermatol 53:201–214
Flatt AE (1948) Refrigerated autogenous skin grafting. Lancet 2:249–251
Flatt AE (1950) Observations on the growth of refrigerated skin grafts. Br J Plast Surg 3:28–33
Flick K (1930) Verfahren zur Entnahme grosser Epidermislappen. Dtsch Z Chir 222:302–305
Gabarro P (1943) A new method of grafting. Br Med J 1:723–724
Gabarro P (1944) Board for cutting skin grafts of definite width. Lancet 2:788
Garlock JH (1933) The full-thickness skin graft, its field of applicability and technical considerations. Ann Surg 97:259–273
Gibson T, Medawar PB (1943) The fate of skin homografts in man. J Anat 77:299–310

Gillies HD, McIndoe AH (1935) The role of plastic surgery in burns due to roentgen rays and radium. Ann Surg 101:979–996
Goode JV (1935) Skin grafting. Ann Surg 101:927–932
Gosset J (1952) Dermatome électrique. Mem Acad Chir 78:145
Hardy SB, McNichol JW (1944) The use of small pieces of film-covered skin grafts. Surg Clin North Am 24:281–292
Howes EL (1947) Topical use of streptomycin in wounds. Am J Med 2:449–456
Humby G (1934) Apparatus for skin graft cutting. Br Med J 1:1078
Humby G (1936) Modified graft-cutting razor. Br Med J 2:1086
Hutchison J, Tough JS, Wyburn GM (1949) Regeneration of sensation in grafted skin. Br J Plast Surg 2:82
Iselin M (1945) Chirurgie de la main. Masson, Paris
Jenney JA (1945) A modification of the plasma fixation method (Sano) of skin grafting by the use of bobbinet and a mirror attachment. Am J Surg 67:3–7
Kernwein GA (1948) Recovery of sensation in split thickness skin grafts. Arch Surg 56: 459–474
Kilner TP (1948) The contracted socket. Trans Ophthalmol Soc UK 67:275–299
Kilner TP, Jackson T (1921) Skin grafting in the buccal cavity. Br J Surg 9:148
Koch SL (1941) The transplantation of skin and subcutaneous tissue to the hand. Surg Gynecol Obstet 72:157
Kredel FE, Evans JP (1933) Recovery of sensation in denervated pedicle and free skin grafts. Arch Neurol Psychiatry 29:1203–1221
Kredel FE, Phemister DB (1939) Recovery of sympathetic nerve function in skin transplants. Arch Neurol Psychiatry 42:403–412
Lagrot F (1947) Présentation d'un rasoir-rabot à greffe réglable. Mem Acad Chir 73:560
Lagrot F (1948) Reflexions sur une série de 100 greffes dermo-épidermiques en vastes lambeaux. Mem Acad Chir 74:110–114
Large A, Heinbecker P (1944) The effect of cooling on wound healing. Ann Surg 120: 727–741
Leithauser DJ (1933) Technic for care of Ollier-Thiersch skin grafts. Ann Surg 97:311–313
Lindquist G (1946) The healing of skin defects. Acta Chir Scand [Suppl 107] 94:1–163
Litton C, Hood GJ (1954) A new giant dermatome. Plast Reconstr Surg 13:240–245
Loeb L (1930) Transplantation and individuality. Physiol Rev 10:547–616
Ludwig FE (1946) The use of acetic acid-glycerin-saline solution in skin grafting. Surgery 19:492–497
MacFee WF (1933) Free full-thickness skin graft: Its field of applicability and technical considerations. Ann Surg 97:616–617
Marcks KM (1943) A modified calibrated skin grafting knife. Milit Surg 92:653–654
Marino H (1948) Improvements and modifications of Padgett's dermatome. Plast Reconstr Surg 3:752–753
Matthews DN (1943) The surgery of repair. Injuries and burns. Thomas, Springfield
Matthews DN (1945) Storage of skin for autogenous grafts. Lancet 1:775–778
May H (1947) Reconstructive and reparative surgery. Davis, Philadelphia
McCaroll HR (1938) The regeneration of sensation in transplanted skin. Ann Surg 108: 309–320
McGregor IA (1950) The regeneration of sympathetic activity in grafted skin as evidenced by sweating. Br J Plast Surg 3:12
McGregor IA, Conway H (1956) Development of lymph flow from autografts and homografts of skin. Transplant Bull 3:46
McIndoe AH (1937) The applications of cavity grafting with skin. Surgery 1:535–537
McIndoe AH, Banister JB (1938) Operation for the cure of congenital absence of vagina. J Obstet Gynaecol Br Emp 45:490–494
McIndoe A, Franceschetti A (1949) Reciprocal skin homografts in a medico-legal case of familial identification of exchanged identical twins. Br J Plast Surg 2:283
Medawar PB (1941) Sheets of pure epidermal epithelium from human skin. Nature 148:783
Medawar PB (1943) The experimental study of skin grafts. Br Med Bull 1:79

Medawar PB (1944) The behaviour and fate of skin autografts and skin homografts in rabbits. J Anat 78: 176–199
Medawar PB (1945) A second study of the behaviour and fate of skin homografts in rabbits. J Anat 79: 157–176
Meek CP (1958) Successful microdermagrafting using the Meek-Wall micro dermatome. Am J Surg 96: 557–558
Meek CP (1963) Extensive severe burn treated with enzymatic debridement and microdermagrafting. Am Surg 29: 61–64
Meloy WC, Letterman GS (1950) The electro-dermatome. Plast Reconstr Surg 6: 84
Mock HE (1943) Refrigeration anaesthesia in skin grafting. JAMA 122: 597–598
Müller-Meernach O (1942) Eine Erleichterung zur Herstellung der Thiersch'schen Läppchen. Muench Med Wochenschr 89: 591
Padgett EC (1932) Is skin grafting with isografts or homografts practicable. Surg Gynecol Obstet 25: 786
Padgett EC (1937) Care of the severely burned with special reference to skin grafting. Arch Surg 35: 64–86
Padgett EC (1942) Skin grafting from a personal and experimental viewpoint. Thomas, Springfield
Padgett EC (1946) Indications for determination of the thickness for split skin grafts. Am J Surg 72: 683–693
Pontén B (1960) Grafted skin. Acta Chir Scand [Suppl] 257: 1–78
Rawles BW (1945) A routine for early skin grafting of deep burns. Surgery 18: 696–706
Reese JD (1946) Dermatape: a new method for the management of split skin grafts. Plast Reconstr Surg 1: 98
Roberts WM, Schaubel HJ (1945) Vaseline gauze contact fixation of split thickness (Padgett) skin grafts. Am J Surg 67: 16–22
Robinson DW (1948) Two improvements for the dermatome. Plast Reconstr Surg 3: 621
Robinson DW (1949) Blood loss from donor sites in skin grafting procedures. Surgery 25: 105–109
Roegholt MN (1976) Vrije huid-transplantatie. (Free skin grafting) in Dutch. Ned Tijdschr Geneesk 120: 398
Rous P (1946) The activation of skin grafts. J Exp Med 83: 383–400
Sachs AE, Goldberg SL (1943) Foreskin isografts. Am J Surg 60: 255–259
Sano ME (1943 a) Skin grafting, a new method based on the principles of tissue culture. Am J Surg 61: 105–106
Sano ME (1943 b) A coagulum contact method of skin grafting as applied to human grafts. Surg Gynecol Obstet 77: 510–513
Schattner A (1944) Report of isograft transplants in identical twins. Arch Otolaryngol 39: 521–522
Schuchardt K (1949) Die freie Hauttransplantation unter besonderer Berücksichtigung der Verwendung von Epidermis-Kutis-Lappen. Dtsch Zahn- Mund- Kieferheilkd 12: 1
Scothorne RJ, Tough JS (1952) Histochemical studies of human skin autografts and homografts. Br J Plast Surg 5: 161–170
Scothorne RJ, Scothorne AW (1953) Histochemical studies on human skin autografts. J Anat 87: 22–29
Shafiroff BGP (1935) An instrument for skin grafts. Ann Surg 101: 814–815
Shumacker HB (1944) An improved cutting edge for the Padgett dermatome. Surgery 15: 457–459
Singer J (1955) Modifications for cutting split skin grafts. Br J Plast Surg 7: 380–381
Sneep AJ, Folkerts JF, Meyling HA (1959) The rehabilitation of patients with deep burns connected with the recovery of function and sensation of grafted skin areas. Noord-Hollandsche Uitgeversmaatschappÿ, Amsterdam
Strumia MM, Hodge CC (1945) Frozen human skin grafts. Ann Surg 121: 860–865
Szodoray L (1931) The structure of the junction of the epidermis and the corium. Arch Dermatol Syphilol 23: 920–925
Tappeiner S (1947) Ein Fortschritt in der Transplantation nach Thiersch durch Verwendung von Penicillinpuder. Wien Klin Wochenschr 59: 244–245

Webster JP (1944 a) Refrigerated skin grafts. Ann Surg 120:431–449
Webster JP (1944 b) Film-cemented skin grafts. Surg Clin North Am 24:251–280
Webster GV (1945) A simple skin graft knife for general use. Am J Surg 67:569–571
Young F, Favata BV (1944) The fixation of skin grafts by thrombin-plasma adhesion. Surgery 15:378–386
Young F (1944) Skin graft fixation by plasma-thrombin adhesion. Ann Surg 120:450–462
Zintel HA (1945) Resplitting split-thickness grafts with the dermatome; method for increasing field of limited donor sites. Ann Surg 121:1–5

Summary and Conclusion

Chapter 1 presents a survey of attempts to graft skin made before Reverdin ultimately succeeded with his method of grafting. The report that skin grafting had been done for centuries in India made a profound impression in Europe. However, it seems unlikely that free skin grafting was really done in India. Bünger (Marburg, Germany) is usually honoured as the first surgeon to perform a successful skin graft. Bünger used a graft which consisted of skin and subcutis.

Another German surgeon, Dieffenbach, distinguished himself especially with skin grafting experiments on animals. His experiments were later continued by Hanff in Berlin. Hanff was still experimenting when Reverdin, in Paris, reported on his first successful skin graft on a human patient.

Chapter 2 discusses developments in skin grafting during the period 1869–1886. In 1869, the Swiss surgeon Reverdin evolved the first reproducible method of grafting skin. In 1886, Thiersch presented guidelines for skin grafting which were to ensure better results. Reverdin performed grafts with small fragments of skin, with a surface area of 3–4 mm^2. The grafts consisted of epidermis and a layer of corium. Grafting was considered to be indicated for all skin defects which showed no healing or delayed healing. The only prerequisite for the skin defect was that it had to be covered by strong, reddish granulation tissue.

The grafts were taken from several sites, but usually from the inside of the upper arm. The grafts were generally cut with the aid of scissors and forceps, and as a rule without anaesthesia. The size and thickness of the grafts varied rather widely, dependent on the surgeons' wishes. Grafts were often divided into small fragments in order to apply the principle of surface area enlargement: In this way regeneration of epithelium could take place from a longer skin edge. Grafts used on functionally important areas were placed close together in order to obtain a cicatrix of good quality. In functionally less important areas the grafts were spaced further apart.

The principal objective of this type of grafting was to promote epithelialization of the wound by formation of epithelium both from the grafts and from the wound edges. Many surgeons were especially fascinated by the phenomenon that grafting seemed to stimulate epithelialization from the wound edges.

One of the first theories on graft healing was advanced by Lindenbaum (1871).

The value of heterografting was likewise studied, using skin from several animal species such as dogs, rabbits and frogs. Besides negative results, positive findings were also described; yet this type of grafting was used only sparingly.

Although the interest in skin grafting showed a marked decline after 1874, one branch of surgery continued to pay close attention to it: palpebral surgery.

Chapter 3 concerns this application of skin grafts to eyelids. Skin grafting continued to play an important role in surgery of the eyelids, and especially in corrections of ectropion, e.g. as a complication of palpebral burns. For reconstruction of eyelids, full-thickness skin grafts were mostly used. The first successful attempt was probably made by the Englishman Lawson (1870). The principle was subsequently adopted in many other countries. In some cases the skin defect resulting from excision of scar tissue was repaired with small grafts in a mosaic pattern. In other cases, one or two larger grafts were used to repair the defect. It is difficult to estimate the true value of the results obtained in palpebral reconstruction, because in many cases the evaluation had to be made when the patient was discharged from hospital.

Not infrequently, discussions of palpebral reconstruction raised the question of whether grafts had to be applied to a fresh wound or to a wound covered by granulations. Surgeons who preferred to delay grafting for a few days thus prevented blood from accumulating beneath the graft. Some surgeons tried to prevent accumulation of blood beneath the graft by making multiple incisions in it, which ensured adequate drainage.

One of the major problems in eyelid surgery was contraction in the graft area, which destroyed the effect of the operation. Skin grafts were used, not only in ectropion but also in other palpebral affections such as trichiasis, and in fresh wounds.

The first suggestions for early excision of burns followed by grafting were made by surgeons who dealt with burns in the palpebral region.

Chapter 4 describes the use of split-skin grafts, full-thickness skin grafts and homografts and heterografts during the period from about 1886 to 1900. The paper read by Thiersch (1886) at a meeting of the German Association of Surgeons caused a sensation and restored skin grafting to a more prominent place in the treatment of various skin defects. Thiersch formulated a number of rules which made skin grafting a standardized procedure. He advised that skin grafts be applied only to a fresh wound bed. Granulation tissue, if present, should be removed. He preferred split-skin autografts and covered the entire skin defect with grafts in order to prevent the contraction which followed grafting by the Reverdin method.

Skin grafts were applied to a variety of skin defects: burns, ulcers and defects which resulted from reconstructive surgery for contractures or congenital anomalies. The grafts were cut with a razor, and those cut by Thiersch measured about 10×2 cm. The skin was stretched and flattened by the hand of an assistant in order to facilitate cutting.

Initially, grafting was as a rule done without anaesthesia, but gradually anaesthesia was used more. The Thiersch principles were at first strictly followed, but over the years they were more and more ignored. One of the first principles to be abandoned was removal of the granulation tissue.

The thickness of split-skin grafts varied rather widely. Surgeons used grafts which comprised only epidermis and the top of the papillary layer, but also grafts which consisted of epidermis and a large thickness of corium. Wound dressings were nearly always applied after grafting, but around the turn of the century, when open wound care became popular, grafted wounds were also increasingly left without dressing. Grafting results were interpreted rather varyingly. Grafting initially seemed a good therapy for ulcers of the leg, but it was later found that the ulcers relapsed about six months after the operation.

Return of sensibility was scarcely considered in the evaluation of results. Goldmann (1894) was one of the first to study return of sensibility in grafts which proved to occur in patches and not to be diffuse. The histological aspects of graft healing were also studied. It was unanimously agreed that the fluid between wound floor and graft was important for the nutrition of the graft. Signs of degeneration developed in the epidermis 3–4 days after grafting, and the superficial layer of epidermis became detached.

Once the circulation in the graft was restored, the rete Malpighi resumed the production of cells. The ectodermal components of hair follicles and sweat glands showed the greatest activity in the production of epithelial cells. How the vascular communication between wound bed and graft was restored, however, remained an enigma.

Skin preservation was also studied in the last decades of the 19th century. It was found that skin had to be kept in a moist environment if it were to retain its regenerative power. Some investigators wondered whether skin could perhaps be better stored at low temperatures than at room temperature. New attempts to make increasing use of epithelial scrapings for grafting were disappointing because the quality of the scars was poor.

Full-thickness skin grafts were hardly used outside the field of eyelid surgery. Von Esmarch pointed out that these grafts merited more extensive use. In subsequent years, Krause made himself famous in the field of full-thickness skin grafting. He preferred these grafts to split-skin grafts because much better results were obtained with them. However, the demands made on technique and wound bed were higher than with other grafting techniques. Surprisingly, homografting was done more frequently with full-thickness skin grafts than with split-skin grafts. This was probably explained by the desire to spare the patient ugly scars in the donor area. In some cases, full-thickness skin grafts measuring no less than 45×7–8 cm were cut.

The healing of full-thickness skin grafts was carefully studied. Signs of regeneration were observed in epidermis and corium within two days. A correlation was found to exist between graft thickness and survival of cellular elements: the thicker the graft, the less favourable the chance of survival of these elements. Some form of circulation between wound bed and graft was demonstrable within three days. The circulation was restored completely in 13 days.

In spite of many negative results with homografts and heterografts, homografting continued to be performed on patients. The results were poor. Publications with case reports on heterografting are so incomplete that the data can hardly be analysed; some of these publications even maintained that good results had been obtained with frog skin.

Beresowsky (1893) studied the healing of frog skin and demonstrated that, in mammals, frog skin grafts played a passive role and merely gave rise to a foreign body reaction.

Chapter 5 discusses the use of skin grafts during the period from about 1900 to about 1930 (the period around the First World War). During the first two decades of the 20th century, skin grafting lost much of its popularity. Nevertheless, there were several important developments during that period. For example, a new range of indications for skin grafting was found: the epithelial inlay. The epithelial inlay could be used to create or to enlarge epithelium-lined cavities.

Other aspects, such as changes in pigmentation and return of sensibility, were still scarcely considered in the evaluation of results. The healing of full-thickness skin grafts received more attention than that of split-skin grafts. The Americans, particularly, were very active in this respect. As already pointed out, little use was made of skin grafts during the first two decades of the 20th century. This was due to disappointing results (probably because the Thiersch principles were ignored). A search for safer procedures commenced, and it is not so surprising that many surgeons reverted to older techniques, with a better chance of graft healing.

The (modified) Reverdin method was rediscovered almost simultaneously in several countries, and one of its staunchest advocates was the American Davis (1914). As in Reverdin's days, grafts were again applied to granulating skin defects. The technique was simple and the chance of healing excellent. The cosmetic results were decidedly poor. Scar contraction occurred even after application of "small deep grafts".

Although in the literature it seemed to have been convincingly demonstrated that homografts could only give a brief transient impression of healing, attempts to achieve permanent healing were made again and again. One of the questions studied was whether skin homografting might be more successful when donor and recipient had the same blood group. Although some investigators believed this to be the case, their observations were later found to be erroneous. Only gradually did investigators come to understand why homografting failed repeatedly. Underwood (1914) suspected a correlation between the clinical conditions of patients treated repeatedly by homografting and anaphylactic reactions. Holman (1925) thought it more likely that the rejection of homografts after 10–12 days and the associated clinical symptoms were the result of an immunity reaction. Subsequently, several investigators carried out experiments in which attempts were made to prevent rejection by blockage of the reticulo-endothelial system.

Chapter 6 outlines developments in skin grafting during the period from about 1930 to about 1950. The evolution of the preceding period was continued during the period around the Second World War. During the war, burns and other types of traumatic skin loss were a very important indication for skin grafting. Epithelial inlays and onlays were given a permanent place in the armamentarium of the plastic surgeon.

The principal developments concerned the technique of skin grafting. The instruments with which the operations were performed were markedly improved. Names still attached to various instruments today date back to this period. British and American surgeons in particular devoted much attention to perfecting instruments and improving techniques.

The healing of skin graft donor sites was studied under various conditions, e.g. when exposed to cold. The influence of various types of dressing on wound healing was likewise studied. Skin was preserved in various ways, both at refrigerator temperature (about 4 °C) and at much lower temperatures. Since the healing of skin grafts continued to show various disturbances, intensive efforts were made to find ways to enhance the adhesion between graft and wound bed so that accumulation of fluid might be prevented and the chances of undisturbed healing improved.

In the evaluation of grafting results, attention was no longer confined to healing and contraction but also focused on such aspects as skin pattern, pigmentation, sensibility and sympathetic functions. Moreover, various experiments were carried out in order to gain a more profound insight into the healing of various types of graft; for example, the healing of pure epidermal grafts was studied.

Homografts again attracted more attention, not as substitutes for autografts but as a temporary integument or a biological dressing, used for example to help patients with large burns through the critical period. Efforts to determine why homografting failed were continued and with success! Gibson and Medawar in particular distinguished themselves with a description of the fate of homografts in patients on the basis of a systematic study. The rejection of homografts proved to result from a systemic reaction, provoked by the antigenic characteristics of homografts. The higher the quantity of the homograft applied, the stronger the subsequent reaction. This reaction was also intensified by repeated grafting of skin from the same donor. Homografting was found to cause active immunization.

In the course of more than a hundred years, skin grafting has become a standard procedure in surgery. The indications for the several types of grafting have become rather uniform. The technical aids at the operations only differ in details. Especially the vast experience gained in World War II provided the opportunity to develop the technique of skin grafting and so the evolution of present day plastic surgery. However, virtually every step in the field of indications, selection of grafts, technique and postoperative care has been based on empiricism. The contribution of research has been small. Yet it is necessary that research should come to play a revolutionary, decisive role in the future to make skin homografting clinically applicable. Although certain technical improvements may still be developed, the answer to the problems of skin homografting will be found in the field of immunology.

Free Skin Grafting Today and Tomorrow

Tom Gibson

I have been interested in the history of free skin grafting for many years and have spoken and written about it on many occasions yet Dr. Klasen has unearthed much material about which I was unaware. His thesis does not make a completely coherent story in which one discovery logically leads on to the next but it illustrates how a volume of knowledge grew and was absorbed into surgical thought and led to our present appreciation of the art and science of free grafting. It is still partly an "art", which is just another way of saying that we are ignorant of some of the precise scientific facts underlying free skin grafting. With experience one obtaines better takes but becomes more and more aware of the miraculous biological phenomenon which makes free skin grafting possible. The take of a free graft would seem to have no survival property to develop in the course of evolution and yet it takes place and makes modern plastic and reconstructive surgery possible.

It is now possible to transplant any thickness of free skin graft up to full thickness, although in the presence of infection the thinner grafts are more likely to succeed. The disadvantage of full-thickness grafts is that, unless they are small and the secondary defect can be closed directly, it must be covered, in turn, with a split-thickness graft. Full-thickness grafts are, of course, cut with a scalpel but a wide range of instruments is available for cutting split-thickness skin. They are now all equipped with some device to permit only the desired thickness to be cut and are powered variously by hand, electric or pneumatic power. But there were advantages in learning, in days long past, how to cut grafts with an open razor or an unguarded blade like the Blair knife; such skill enabled one to cut quite appreciable pieces of skin with an ordinary scalpel blade. Instruments are available to cut grafts of almost any size required clinically. In the excisional surgery of lymphoedema and the reapplication of degloved skin, large sheets may be needed. The dermatome of Gibson and Ross will cut skin grafts 27 cm broad and any length; Barinka's huge drum dermatome will cut even broader sheets.

Cutting grafts by hand needs a steady sawing movement with the skin under moderate tension. In inexperienced hands the knife will leave ragged, irregular scars along the margin of the donor area and, for this reason, many prefer to use a mechanical instrument which will cut exactly what it is set to do. But the hand-held blade in experienced hands will cut a graft far more quickly and leave a scar as neat.

The method of the application of some free skin grafts has changed in recent years. Immediately after the great expansion of plastic surgery in World War II, it was widely believed and taught that pressure had to be applied to free skin grafts to enable them to take. Ferris Smith in his book *Plastic and Reconstructive Surgery* (Saunders, 1950) actually specified a pressure of 30 mm Hg and designed a pneumatically inflatable rubber bag to apply over full-thickness grafts to the face.

It is now apparent that the tie-over dressing with a bolus of this or that or a bag is not only unnecessary but may be harmful. A stitched-in skin graft with a tie-over dressing is immobile and if it is applied over moving muscles there is a likelihood that the budding vessels will be sheared and ruptured. It is much better in such cases to wait 2 or 3 days until all bleeding has stopped and before granulations are sprouting, and lay the skin graft, cut at the original operation and stored in a refrigerator, on the defect. A bandage may be applied for social reasons but not to apply pressure; more often the grafted area is left exposed. In my Unit this technique of delayed grafting has been the lazy (or perhaps, busy) plastic surgeon's method. The grafts are applied in the wards by the nursing staff who enjoy doing it and do it well! It is realised, however, that this would not be acceptable in some other countries. There is no doubt that such delayed, unpressurized grafts take well and are, of course, immune from the risks of haematomas.

With thicker grafts, i.e. full-thickness and composite grafts, I feel that pressure dressings should be used. Blood may enter such grafts, drift to the peripheral vessels, stagnate and never circulate. Slight pressure to prevent over-dilatation of the capillaries would seem to be worthwhile, but this is "art" rather than "science".

The use of homograft (allograft) skin is well established in the treatment of extensive deep burns. The skin may be obtained from fresh cadavers and stored for some days in a refrigerator, or kept for many weeks by freezing in liquid nitrogen. In extensive burns the immune reaction is depressed and homograft skin will usually remain in situ for 3–4 weeks. Tissue typing and matching the skin with that of the patient may make longer survival possible but seems hardly necessary, except in special cases. The homografts, after rejection, may be replaced with autografts; a useful technique is to alternate narrow strips of homograft and autograft, so that when the homograft dies the autograft will grow out and cover the defect which it occupied. Immunosuppression has no place in skin homografting.

What then of the future? The technique of free skin autografting is so reliable that I would see little advancement in techniques over those already available. The use of free flaps transferred by microvascular anastomoses may make free skin grafts less appropriate but they will still be widely used. It is possible, but unlikely, that the immune response to homografting will be overcome but my Protestant upbringing rejects any idea of one individual permanently wearing another's skin.

D. L. Ballantyne, J. M. Converse

Experimental Skin Grafts and Transplantation Immunity

A Recapitulation

1979. 60 figures. XIX, 192 pages
ISBN 3-540-90425-5

Contents: Vascularization of Skin Grafts: Autografts and Allografts. – Acute Rejection of First-Set Allografts. – Chronic Reaction Patterns of First-Set Skin Allografts. – Reaction Patterns of Skin Xenografts. – Role of the Dosage Phenomenon in Allograft and Xenograft Reactions. – Behavior of Preserved Skin Grafts in Their Hosts. – Survival and Rejection of Second-Set Skin Allografts. – References. – Index.

Allografts have long been used as investigative tools in transplantation research. Because of the skin's high antigenicity, skin grafts are the most frequently used research material. The achievement of the permanent survival of skin allografts is felt to be the final solu
to acceptance problems in allografts of other tissues. This monograph provides transplantation researchers with a review of the significant literature covering clinical and experimental research into various types of orthotopic skin grafts transplanted to normal recipients. The nature of reparative changes, including graft vascularization, is described, as are biologic events that determine the behavior and eventual fate of such grafts after transplantation. Also discussed are diagnostic assay procedures used to establish criteria for graft behavior and survival endpoints, and to support theories underlying the immune mechanisms responsible for graft rejection.
This book will be of interest to physicians and researchers in the fields of reconstructive plastic surgery, tissue and organ transplantation and the immunobiology of transplantation, as well as to scientists in cryobiology and experimental biology.

Springer-Verlag
Berlin
Heidelberg
New York